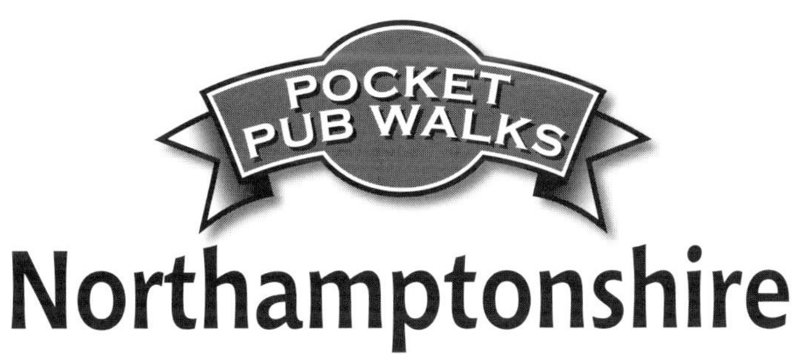

Northamptonshire

Judith & Ron Smith

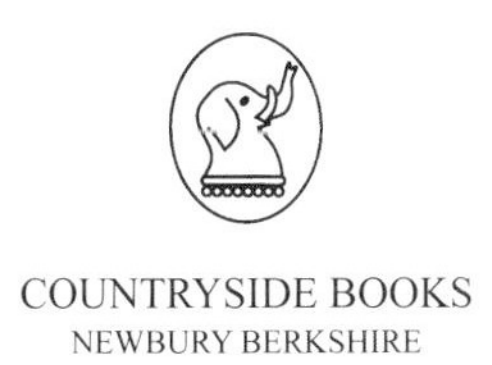

COUNTRYSIDE BOOKS
NEWBURY BERKSHIRE

First published 2008

COUNTRYSIDE BOOKS
3 Catherine Road
Newbury, Berkshire

To view our complete range of books,
please visit us at
www.countrysidebooks.co.uk

ISBN 978 1 84674 084 8

Photographs by Ron Smith
Photo of the Butcher's Arms on page 76
courtesy of Alan Newman
Maps by Gelder Design & Mapping
Designed by Nautilus Design

Produced through MRM Associates Ltd, Reading
Printed by Cambridge University Press

Contents

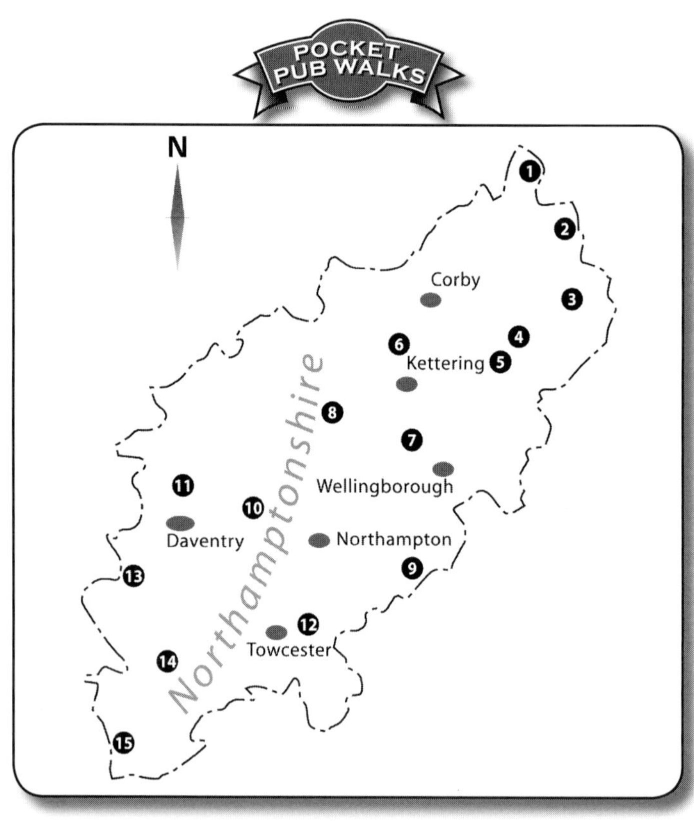

Area map showing location of the walks

Introduction

With simple beauty born of lovely grace,
Our County lanes a tender welcome give
The thoughtful wanderer, who loves to trace
The open book of nature's narrative.

George Harrison, Northamptonshire poet, (1876-1950).

In compiling this book of walks we have endeavoured to spread them throughout the county. Usefully, the M1 and the A6 roads, running north-south, divide the area into thirds, thus allowing approximately five walks in each area.

Northamptonshire is a long county, approximately 70 miles north to south, and 20 miles at its widest. Lying as it does in the centre of England, it comprises countryside that is passed through by many but investigated by few. Bounded by no fewer than nine other counties, it has getting on for 2,000 miles of footpaths, byways and bridleways. Traditionally it is the county of spires and squires – with the spires mainly in the east and the houses of the squires scattered throughout.

Numerous natural and man-made routes have criss-crossed the area since prehistoric times, from the limestone ridge that is now the Jurassic Way to the Roman Watling and Ermine streets, and then to the canals, roads and railways of more recent times. Who would think such delightful walking is to be enjoyed in close proximity to the Watford Gap? Six rivers rise in Northamptonshire and have been used and modified by man to transport goods, to irrigate the countryside and to provide a much used leisure facility.

The county is blessed with rich agricultural land much sought after by royalty and sundry other landowners, who were also attracted by the marvellous hunting country. Charles I even had a break from the pressing matters of state to hunt in the north of the county during the Civil War. These landowners contributed to the countryside's rich architectural heritage, as reflected in the castles and mansions, churches and monuments scattered throughout this part of England.

Wildlife abounds. Being on the flight path of migrating birds, many interesting species are to be seen on the walks, together with such residents as the red kite, buzzards and an abundance of smaller birds. Keeping one's eyes open will often be rewarded by glimpses of deer, foxes, signs of an occasional badger, the ubiquitous rabbit and many other small animals – even the occasional walker.

Come and enjoy.

Judith & Ron Smith

Publisher's Note

We hope that you obtain considerable enjoyment from this book; great care has been taken in its preparation. However, changes of landlord and actual closures are sadly not uncommon. Likewise, although at the time of publication all routes followed public rights of way or permitted paths, diversion orders can be made and permissions withdrawn.

We cannot, of course, be held responsible for such diversion orders and any inaccuracies in the text which result from these or any other changes to the routes nor any damage which might result from walkers trespassing on private property. We are anxious though that all details covering the walks and pubs are kept up to date and would therefore welcome information from readers which would be relevant to future editions.

The simple sketch maps that accompany the walks in this book are based on notes made by the author whilst checking out the routes on the ground. However, for the benefit of a proper map, we do recommend that you purchase the relevant Ordnance Survey sheet covering your walk. The Ordnance Survey maps are widely available, especially through booksellers and local newsagents.

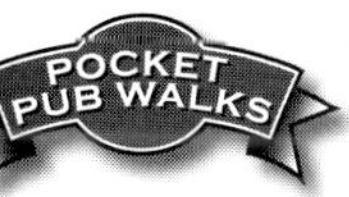

1 Easton on the Hill

The Oak Inn

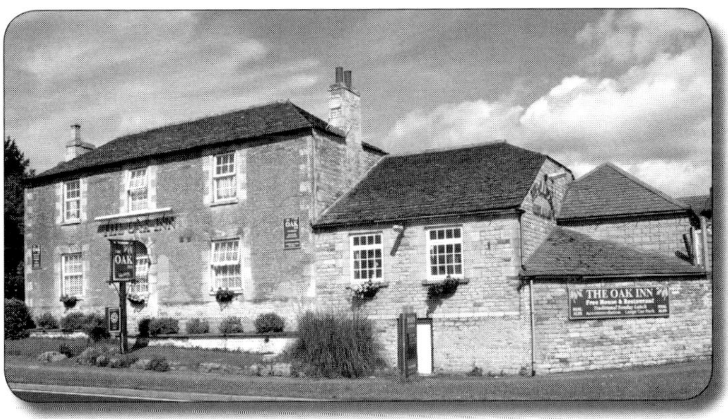

The village of Easton on the Hill is a feast for the eyes! Stone cottages with their roofs of slate from nearby Collyweston tumble down the hill into the Welland valley. Over forty of these houses are listed, the oldest, apart from the 12th-century church, is the early 16th-century Priest's House, which was restored by the National Trust. Captain Skynner who lived in the 300-year-old Glebe House, was captain of the *Lutein* whose bell is kept at Lloyd's in London and rung when a ship is lost at sea.

The walk takes you through the winding streets of this amazing village and on through water meadows by the River Welland with a panoramic view of Stamford as you go. After touching the edge of Stamford, it returns through shady woodland and along a bridleway to Easton.

Distance – 4½ miles.

OS Explorer 234 Rutland Water. GR 011040.

Starting point The Oak Inn, which sits on the main Kettering to Stamford road. There is plenty of parking for customers at the rear of the inn. Otherwise park in Porter's Lane beside the pub.

How to get there *Easton on the Hill is 2 miles south of Stamford on the A43 Kettering road.*

THE PUB The **Oak Inn** is an imposing building of mellow stone at the southern end of the village. It has a comfortable bar area as well as a conservatory where food is served. Light snacks, including sandwiches with a wide range of fillings, are available. Pies, breaded plaice, Mediterranean chicken and venison could be on offer along with seasonal dishes, to be followed by delicious desserts. This is a free house with a good selection of beers, among them Grainstore Rutland Panther, Ruddles, Greene King and assorted lagers.

Food is served on Tuesday to Saturday from 12 noon to 2 pm and 6.30 pm to 9 pm and on Sunday from 12 noon to 2.30 pm. The pub is closed on Mondays.
☎ *01780 752286*

1 Take **Porter's Lane**, which runs down beside the pub into the village. Modern housing soon gives way to Collyweston-roofed stone cottages. Turn right into **The Lane** and then left into **Church Street**, noticing a wonderful free-standing fig tree in a garden on your right just before a footpath sign (not yours!). Carry straight on, passing the Norman **church of All Saints**.

2 After the large institute on the right, turn right onto a footpath signed as the **Jurassic Way**. Cross a bark-strewn path to a stile and follow the markers, which are also marked '**Hereward Way**'. Turn left over a stile in the hedge and carry on diagonally across the field towards some telegraph poles with **Stamford** in view straight ahead. Emerge onto a wide double rutted grass track, keeping left. This can be rather muddy, being overhung with oak and sycamore trees. As you leave the track, head for a marker at the bottom right-hand corner of the field.

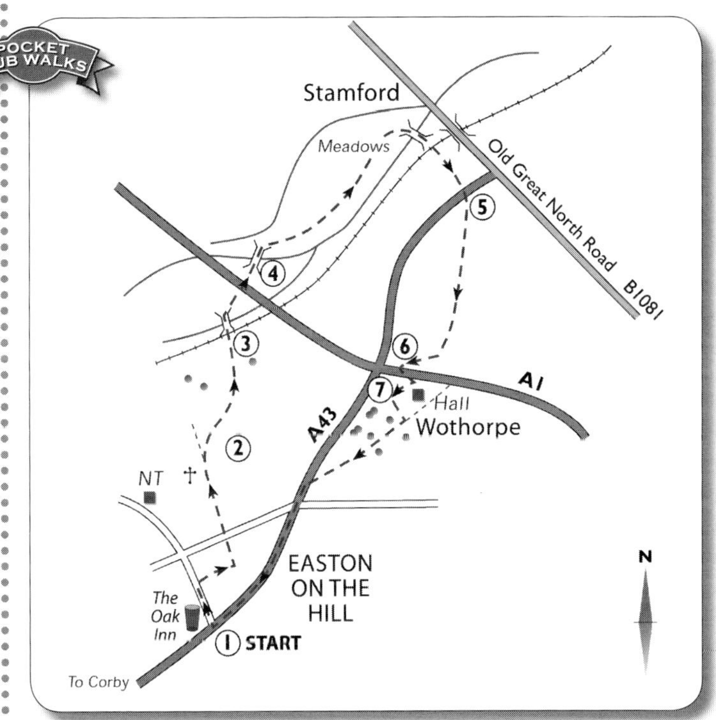

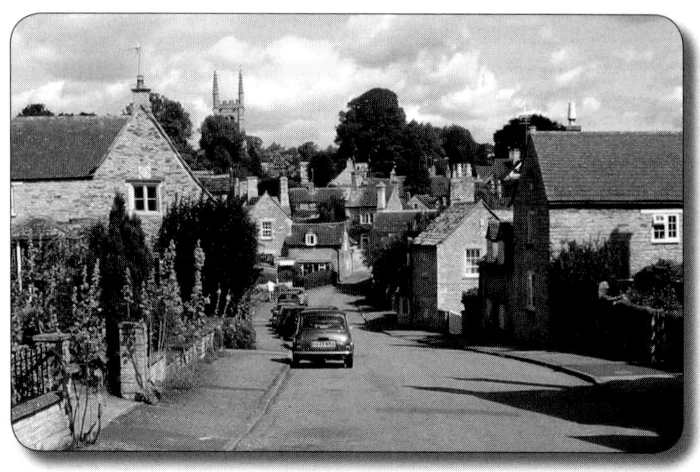

The mellow stone colours of Easton on the Hill.

3 Go over a wooden plank bridge and up the steps to the railway line, taking heed of the warning signs. Continue on over another wooden bridge and veer right to a gap in the hedge leading under the A1. Enter a wide meadow with the river running swiftly on the left. This is a lovely spot with copious wild flowers in season, seeds blowing about and butterflies enjoying the breeze.

4 Turn left over a metal bridge; linger awhile to count the churches with their towers and spires. Follow the well signed path and where it divides keep right towards a stone monument commemorating Boudicca's pursuit of the 9th Roman legion across the river. Walk straight ahead under the overhead wires to a wooden gate into **Stamford meadows** and very soon join the path and turn right over a metal gate leading to a car park. Carry straight on up **Wothorpe Road** to the A43. Glance to the right to see an interesting row of cottages called **Friar's Callis**.

5 Cross the A43 to a footpath sign. Go straight ahead on the **Lincolnshire Way**, keeping a stock fence on your left. Cross a footbridge and go through a kissing gate to walk across the centre of the field towards a wooden bridge, which leads to a narrow path hedged with holly. Emerge onto a road, cross over and continue down a cul de sac, with **Parrish House** on the left, to a footpath, bottom left. Climb a stile and aim for a large ash tree in the top left-hand corner of the field. Go over the stile and keep straight ahead with the hedge on your right.

Place of interest nearby

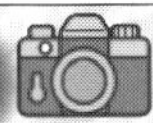

The **Priest's House** (National Trust) is a lovely looking dwelling built around 1500. As the name would suggest, it was built for celibate clergy of the time and is a rare example of a pre-Reformation house. After becoming a barn, it was rescued from demolition by The Peterborough Society. It contains a small and interesting museum illustrating past village life.

☎ *01780 762619. The house is unmanned but names of key holders are on the property's notice board. The House is well signed off the main road.*

The conservation town of **Stamford** itself – a Mecca for film makers – is well worth a visit. Like Easton, it is rich in delightful stone buildings, which here are rather more formal.

Burghley, just outside the town on the B1443, is the 'largest and grandest Elizabethan house in the country'. It is now known mostly for the horse trials that take place in September, but the house contains wonderful treasures and the parkland, landscaped by Capability Brown, is beautiful. There is a very good restaurant in the Orangery.

☎ *01780 752451.*

At the end of the field veer right as signed. The A1 runs behind the hedge on the left but look the other way for a good view of **Stamford**.

6 Turn left under the A1 and keep up left to a footpath sign. Turn sharp right. After a small stone barn, you will come across a delightful duck sanctuary with a pond; though it says 'welcome', you may have difficulty getting past the padlock! The ruins of **Wothorpe Hall** can be seen clearly on the left. The hall was built in the 17th century for Thomas Cecil, Earl of Exeter, who was Lord Burghley's eldest son; it has been in ruins since the 18th century.

7 Carry on to the top left-hand corner of the field onto a track and across to join the path which states that it has been recently diverted. This is a wide grassy track with new hedge planting on either side and a very large building undergoing considerable renovation on the left. Go through a gate and turn right onto a bridleway into woodland. Soon a long track with butterflies dancing in front of you in the summer months leads ultimately to the A43 again, at which point turn left to **Easton** and the **Oak Inn**.

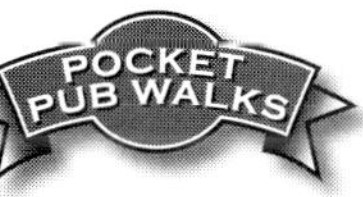

2 Nassington

The Black Horse

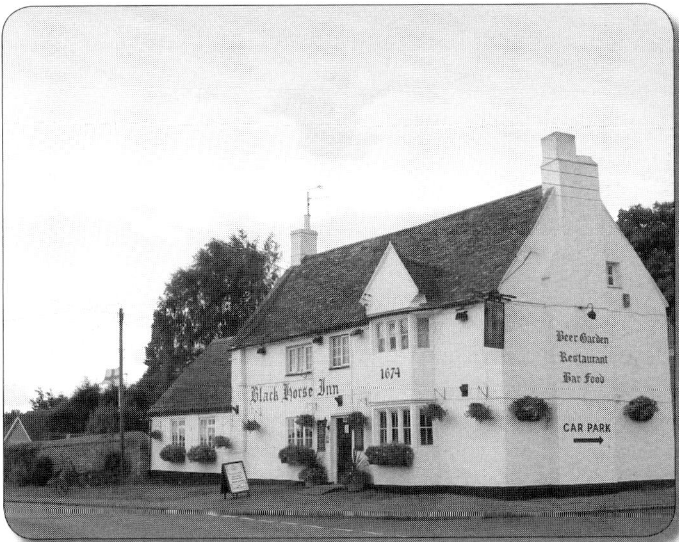

The village of Nassington, so full of picturesque houses, has obviously been a busy place for centuries. Early workings show remains of Roman occupation, and a large and important Anglo-Saxon cemetery discovered in 1942 was found to contain shields and spears, which might suggest that warriors lived here. The 13th-century Prebendal Manor House is thought to be the earliest surviving manor in the country. It is a private

Distance – 5 miles.

OS Explorer 227 Peterborough. GR 066961.

Starting point The Black Horse at Nassington where, with permission, customers may leave their cars while they walk. Otherwise park alongside the road in the village.

How to get there *Take the A605 between Thrapston and the A1 near Peterborough. Turn off 2 miles north of Oundle, on the road signed to Fotheringhay, from where, opposite the church, you follow signs to Nassington. The Black Horse is on the left as you enter the village.*

dwelling today but open to the public in the summer months, along with the medieval garden, and has 'event' days, one of which brought the BBC and Alan Titchmarsh to the village!

This walk, full of interest, takes you to a mill, through beautiful water meadows and into the Old Sulehay Forest, which is a Site of Special Scientific Interest with its lovely birch trees and wildlife. A sidestep over the magnificent packhorse bridge into the village of Wansford with its Haycock Hotel is well worth taking.

THE PUB

The **Black Horse** has stood in Nassington since 1674 though it has changed somewhat since! It is a busy pub with a cosy bar area and the fireplace from Fotheringhay Castle where Mary Queen of Scots ended her days. Good basic fare is on offer here with a comprehensive snack menu alongside meat, fish and vegetarian dishes. There are some impressive desserts. Beers include Pigs Do Fly from the Pot Belly Brewery, Kettering, Draught Mild from Earl of Soham Brewery, Woodbridge, Black Sheep from Yorkshire, guest ales and assorted lagers.

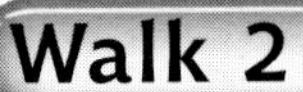

Food is served every day from 12 noon to 3 pm and 6 pm to 9 pm.
☎ *01780 782324*

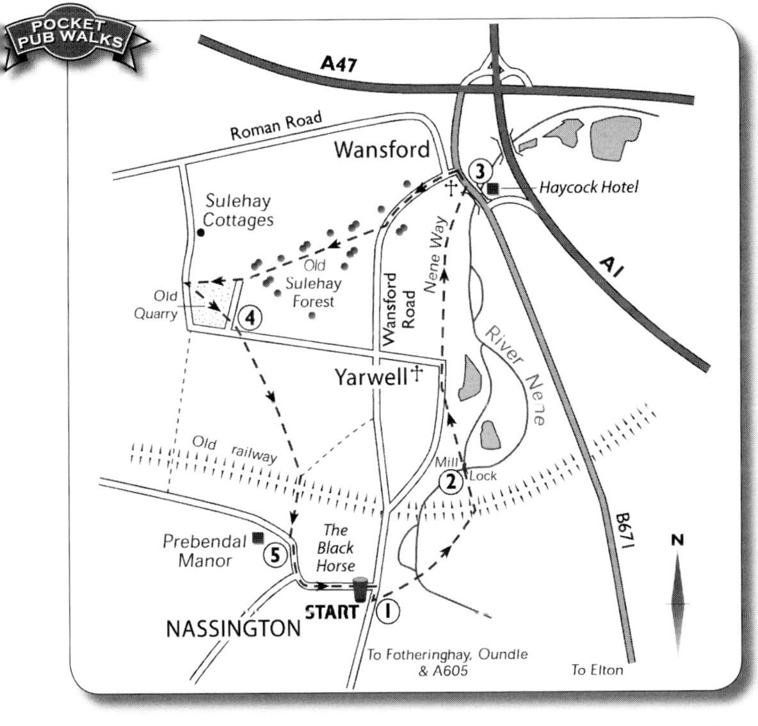

There is plenty to see in **Fotheringhay village**. The imposing church of St Mary and All Saints with its flying buttresses and lantern tower was once the centrepiece of a large college (a wonderful scale model is on view inside) and contains memorials to Edward, 2nd Duke of York, and Richard, 3rd Duke of York, erected by Elizabeth I. The remains of the castle sit sadly by the River Nene; its stone was spread around the vicinity and the Scottish connection is maintained in the abundance of thistles around the site. They are known as 'Mary's tears' and were often sown near houses she inhabited.

1 On leaving the **Black Horse**, turn right into **Fotheringhay Road** and take the footpath on the left. This is the **Nene Way**, which will lead you to **Yarwell Mill**. The original route took you across some stepping stones, but a sign now leads straight ahead at that point so as to avoid a ducking! Shortly, step right onto the bridge for a moment to enjoy watching the sparkling river as it rushes beneath the overhanging trees, before continuing on the path.

2 On arriving at the mill, busy with boats, cross the lock and, with the mill house in front of you, turn left to a red and white barrier. When you emerge on the road, take a **Nene Way** sign right leading along the hedge in a large field. Soon there is a sign with two yellow footprints; bear across diagonally to a road at the top and turn right into the village of **Yarwell**, which was once a centre for stonemasons and consequently where there are some lovely cottages and houses. Where the road veers left, carry on down a well signed path with pretty gardens on either side, arriving in a large field with views over the valley. **Simsey Island** is signed here; you might like to take a short detour to visit the largest island in the Nene. Continue following the signs towards **Wansford in England**.

3 Having emerged onto the road over a stile, turn left and left again by the church onto the Yarwell road leading uphill. Shortly after passing a large metal barn, turn right onto a bridleway and into **Old Sulehay Forest**, which is a SSSI. A signboard gives an indication as to what one might hope to see. It is a delight to walk in these woodlands. Carry on along the path, passing a deep, water-filled quarry on the left. Very soon you go through

a gate on the left where you enter the quarry with its abundance of wild flowers in season, low growing shrubs, dog roses and silver birch. Three paths now lie before you and the left-hand one is yours, taking you into spinneys of silver birch. At the second clearing there is a signboard opposite which, on the left, is a gate leading through onto a narrow, rather overhung path, which then opens up before reaching the road.

4 Cross the road and go over a stile into a field, which you cross, then go diagonally left to a waymarker at a gate. Bear diagonally right to another marker, which in turn points you further along the hedge to a sign leading you right towards the spire of **Nassington church**. You continue along grassy paths with larks ascending, until you bear left through a gate onto a bridleway, which is rather rutted. Continue down under a railway bridge to the village of **Nassington**, going straight ahead to the main road.

5 Turn left, walking past **Prebendal Manor House**, to the end of the road and the **Black Horse**.

Place of interest nearby

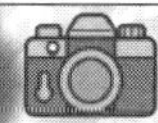

The **Prebendal Manor House** is a good place to go to learn what it was like to live in the Middle Ages. It was the royal manor of King Canute before being passed to the Prebendaries of the church who held it from the 12th century up until 1846. The gardens, complete with 'medieval' gardener, have been lovingly restored and are a joy to visit.
☎ *01780 782575.*

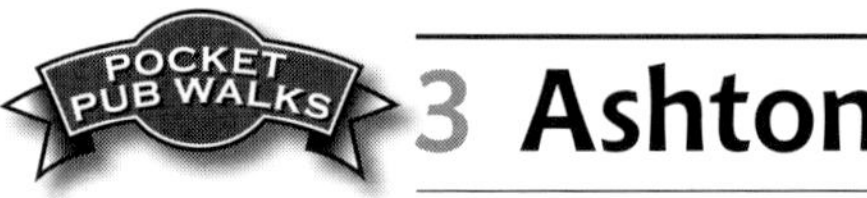

3 Ashton

The Chequered Skipper

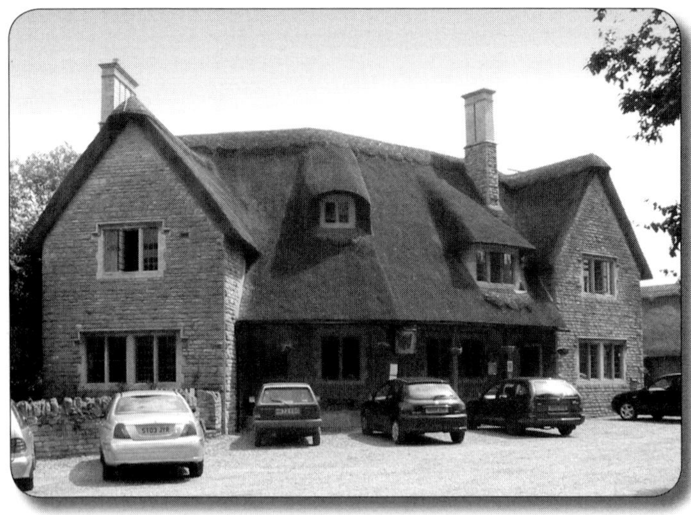

Arriving in this picturesque, quiet village with its large green surrounded by thatched stone cottages and ringed with chestnut trees, you might be forgiven for thinking that nothing could disturb the tranquil scene. How wrong you would be! If 'conkers' is your game, this is your spiritual home. On the Sunday nearest 12th October, thousands descend to enjoy the World Conker Championships, which take place amid great razzmatazz and raise thousands of pounds for the blind. Ashton is an estate village built in 1900 by Charles Rothschild, all of whose cottages were supplied with electricity and water and the luxury, in those days, of a bathroom.

This is an idyllic walk starting in the village, with a brief sortie into Oundle to whet the appetite for a further visit! It continues out into water meadows alongside the Nene and all the beauty it offers. The area is designated as a Site of Special Scientific Interest. The walk stays by the river all the way back to Ashton.

Distance – 3½ miles.

OS Explorer 227 Peterborough. GR 056882.

Starting point The Chequered Skipper. There is plenty of space to park in its environs.

How to get there *At the roundabout on the A605 just north of Oundle take the exit marked 'Ashton 1 mile'. A sign will turn you left into the village and the Chequered Skipper.*

THE PUB

The **Chequered Skipper** is named after a butterfly now extinct in England but happily living in Scotland. The pub has had something of a chequered career having been burnt down in 1996 following a fire in the thatch. Thankfully it has been rebuilt in the same style, matching the charming cottages that ring the green. It has a restaurant and bar area with menus displayed on blackboards and in good weather food can be taken onto the tables on the green. Filled ciabattas, jacket potatoes and ploughman's are among the snacks available, alongside varied dishes such as deep-fried fritter of Brie with cranberry sauce, home-made smoked haddock and salmon fish cakes. There is an assortment of local and national beers and lagers, among them Oakham and Adnam's Southwold ales.

Food is served Monday to Friday 11.30 am to 2 pm and 6 pm to 9.30 pm; Saturday 11.30 am to 2.30 pm and 6 pm to 9.30 pm; and Sunday 12 noon to 3 pm and 6 pm to 9 pm.
☎ *01832 273494*

1 Leave the **Chequered Skipper**, walking diagonally right, and follow the path alongside the wall with the 17th-century chapel and one-time school behind it. Go through the gate into a large field, often full of sheep, and continue in a straight line

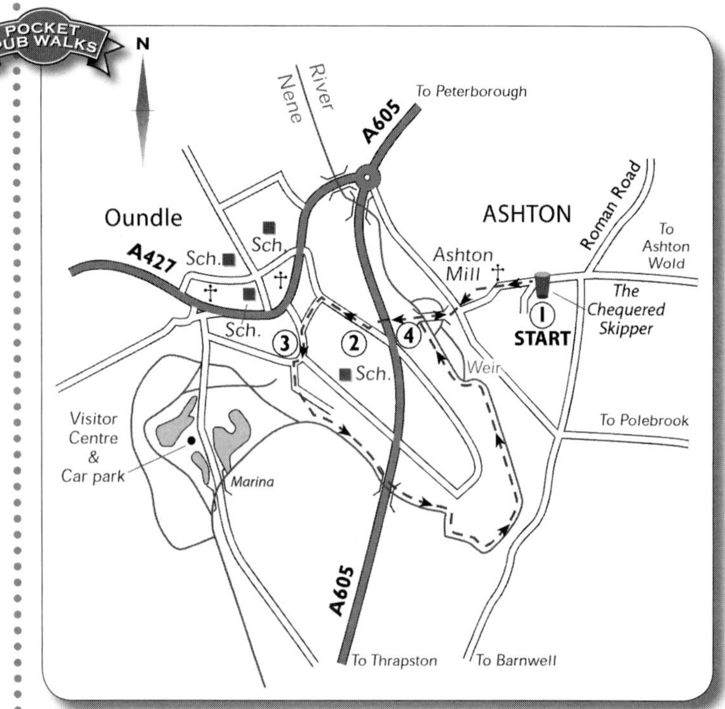

to a sign in the hedge, where you emerge on the road. Cross over, turning right to another sign 50 yards ahead, which will take you left by the now deserted mill. It was from here that Ashton was supplied with water and electricity in 1900. The track leads to a metal bridge. Beyond this, head for the busy A605, which you cross with the greatest care onto a tarmac footpath. Cross a minor service road and continue to the next road.

2 Turn right to a mini roundabout and then left into **East Road**. Follow the road, passing a supermarket on your right, until you reach a pillar box. (A 100-yard detour right at this point will lead you to **Oundle market place** and a cup of coffee!)

3 Turn left at the pillar box and continue on past the end of **Herne Road**, walking straight down a track to a kissing gate beside a metal farm gate. Cross the water meadow, going diagonally left to the river bank, and marvel at the tranquil scene. Many years ago it might not have been so peaceful – you might have come face to face with Mushie the lion! He was a large Abyssinian creature, once part of a circus act, who lived in a wagon alongside his owner's caravan and was brought to the meadows to get his 'greens'. His roar apparently heralded rain and sent the local

Place of interest nearby

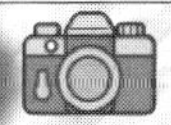

Oundle is a charming stone-built market town watched over by the magnificent 200-year-old crocketed spire of St Peter's church. It has a wealth of interesting buildings, many of them owned by Oundle public school. The town is full of interesting shops and places to eat. The tourist office on West Street near the war memorial will supply a leaflet of a town walk.

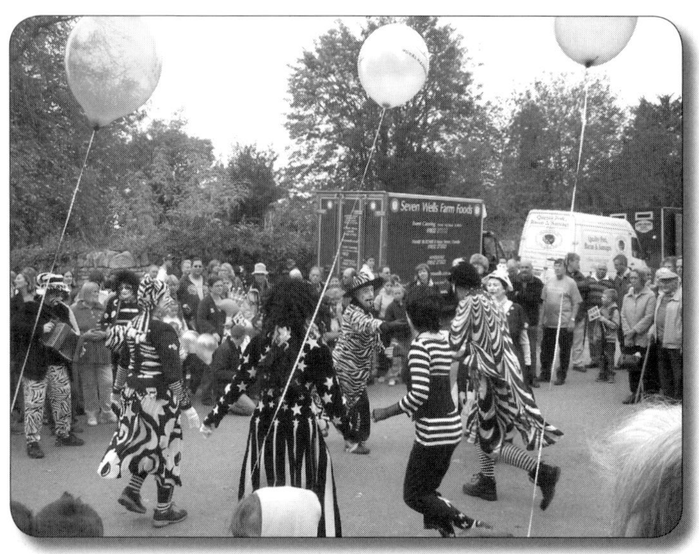

Fun at the World Conker Championships, Ashton.

inhabitants rushing to rescue their washing. The wildlife now is much more benign; gentle cattle come down to drink, heron stand sentinel and in summer water lilies shine at the margins of the river. Keep on the path beside the river, going through many gates, for approximately 2½ miles, giving ample opportunity to admire this beautiful stretch of the **Nene**. The odd boat glides by, the peace only disturbed briefly by the A605, which this time runs overhead. The sound of rushing water tumbling over a weir behind the trees heralds a left turn to a gate leading round the trees and back to the riverbank.

4 Soon the metal bridge over which you came at the start of the walk hoves into view. Cross it and retrace your steps to the mill and thence to the **Chequered Skipper**.

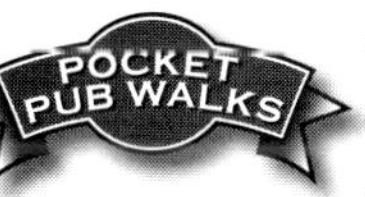

4 Wadenhoe

The King's Head

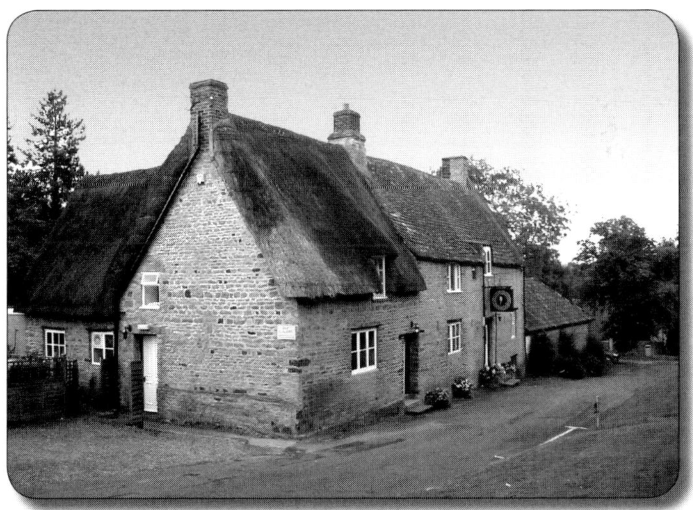

Wadenhoe is one the county's most attractive villages with its limestone buildings roofed with thatch, Collyweston stone and tiles. In the past it was a thriving community with a manor house, large mill, dovecote and alehouse. George Ward Hunt, who lived here whilst Chancellor of the Exchequer in Disraeli's government, installed the first rural telegraph office in order to keep in touch with Whitehall. An enterprising chap, he built his own gasworks to supply the cottages and light the way to his house.

This delightful walk, which follows a section of the Nene Way, passes through one of the largest areas of water meadows in the county, where there is a wonderful variety of flowering plants and wildlife. The route continues on to the 13th-century church of St John the Baptist at Achurch whose churchyard is a mass of snowdrops in early spring. The full circuit visits the village of Pilton before returning to Wadenhoe and the charming King's Head pub in its riverside setting.

Distance – 3½ miles.

OS Explorer 224 Corby, Kettering & Wellingborough. GR 011834.

Starting point The King's Head. Customers may leave their cars in the car park while they walk – please ask first – otherwise there is parking below the pub alongside the village hall.

How to get there *Turn off the A605 between Oundle and Thrapston at Thorpe Waterville. Go through Aldwincle and take the sign right to Wadenhoe. The church and the King's Head are well signposted at the southern end of the village.*

THE PUB

The **King's Head**, a charming old pub in an idyllic spot, started life as an alehouse before the Civil War but has been considerably upgraded since then! It has a very good restaurant area and two bars as well as a terrace overlooking the lawns sloping down to the river. The menu is comprehensive and includes Barnwell Bitter battered haddock, Cumberland sausage and mash, vegetarian options and snacks such as filled rolls and ploughman's. Oakham ales and the local Digfield brew from Barnwell are among the beers on offer.

Food is served from 12 noon to 2.15 pm and 6.15 pm to 9.15 pm on Monday to Saturday and at lunchtime on Sunday.
☎ *01832 720024*

1 Walk up the hill from the **King's Head** and turn right down **Mill Lane**, which becomes a short track leading to a wooden bridge affording a good view of the mill and mill house. Continue on, turning left along the river, signposted '**Nene Way**'. This is the largest area of wet woodland in the county and has a wonderful variety of flowering plants and wildlife; it is a Site of Special Scientific Interest.

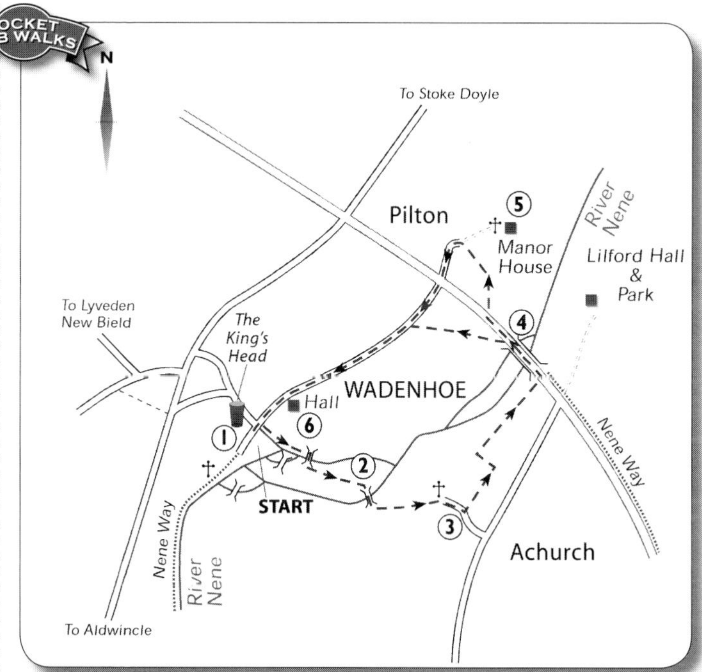

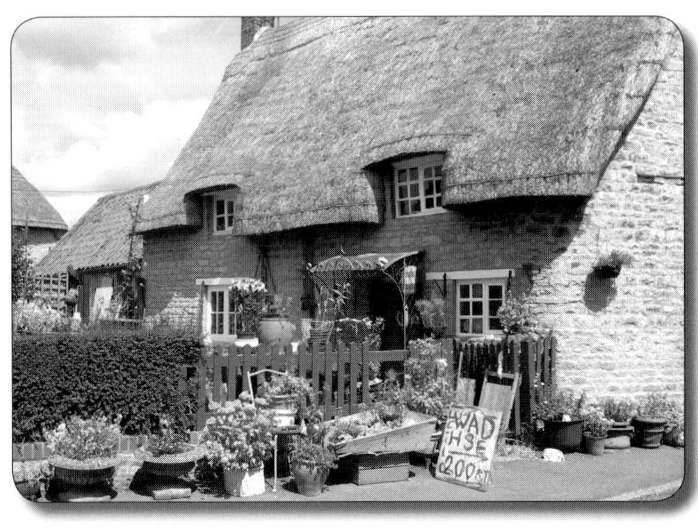

An attractive cottage in Wadenhoe.

2 The path veers right over a raised footbridge then heads left up to the **church of St John the Baptist** at **Achurch**. Go through the kissing gate into the churchyard, which in early spring (or when climate change dictates) is a mass of snowdrops. Walk through the lychgate dedicated to Lord Lilford who is buried along with his wife near the eastern end of the church. He was a renowned ornithologist and the founder of the Natural History Society of Northamptonshire.

3 After reading some interesting history on the wall, continue along the road for about 100 yards. Turn left at the **Nene Way** sign onto a broad track into woodland known as **The Linches**. You will come to a clearing with a Nene Way sign leading you left down some wooden-faced steps onto a narrow path with the river below, which leads you to **Lilford Lock**. On reaching the road, turn left over two bridges.

4 At this point you have two choices. *For a shorter walk,* take the footpath left diagonally across two fields and join the road going left back into **Wadenhoe**, picking up the route at the end of point 5. *To complete the full route,* carry on along the road. When you are level with the 'Single Track' sign facing you, go over a well hidden wooden stile in the hedge on the right into a large field with two magnificent lime trees. Keep to the left of these, going diagonally up the slope and through a metal farm gate into the field above and head for the village of **Pilton**. Turn right along a gravelled track to visit the pretty enclave of **St Mary and All Saints' church**, with a manor house built by the Treshams of Gunpowder Plot fame. Glance to the right to see **Lilford Hall**, an imposing edifice with an amazing array of chimneys.

5 Turn back to **Pilton village**, noticing as you follow the road the **Old Watch House** on the left with its bellflower frieze and strange look-out like a chimney with a pyramid roof. At the road junction cross over and follow the road for ¾ mile back to **Wadenhoe**.

6 You will pass **Wadenhoe House** and beyond it a dovecote, built during the Napoleonic Wars. At the road junction either take a few steps right to view the old 'post office telegraph' sign or turn left and walk down the hill to return to the **King's Head**.

Place of interest nearby

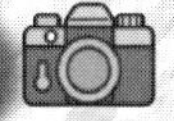

Barnwell Country Park, just off the A605 south of Oundle, is an area of meadows, lakes and marshland for all ages to enjoy. There is also an award-winning visitor centre, which is open at weekends and bank holidays. ☎ *01832 273435.*

5 Lowick

The Snooty Fox

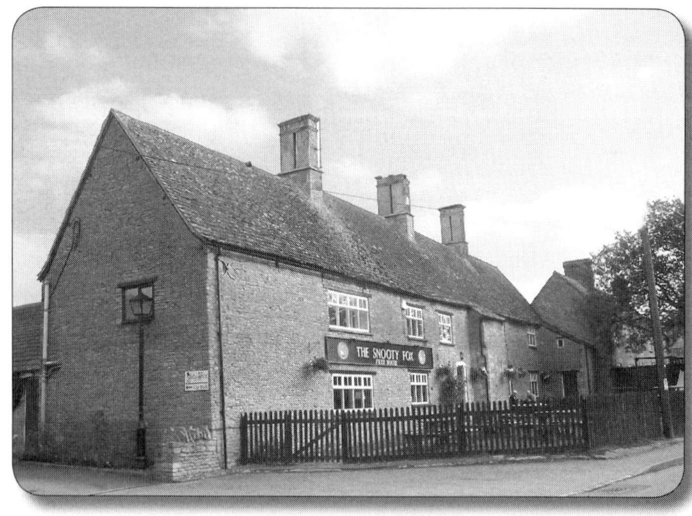

Lowick's quiet roads are lined with stone cottages watched over by St John's church with its elaborately pinnacled lantern tower (the key holder's name is in the porch). A quite lovely alabaster tomb lies within depicting a knight and his lady holding hands. Much of the land and many of the houses are owned by the Drayton Estate and the main house stands in beautiful parkland at the end of Drayton Road. The house is a wonderfully romantic-looking building of turrets and battlements; it was built originally around 1300 and has never been sold or let since! It is not open to the public other than by appointment.

This is a walk through lovely countryside rich in wildlife, with a visit to the pretty villages of both Sudborough and Slipton, not to mention passing in front of the splendid Drayton House set in beautiful pastures.

Distance – 5½ miles.

OS Explorer 224 Corby, Kettering & Wellingborough. GR 978807.

Starting point The Snooty Fox. With permission customers may leave their cars in the large car park while they are walking; otherwise park at the roadside.

How to get there *From junction 12 of the A14 take the A6116 Corby road. Go left at the first turn for Lowick. The Snooty Fox is on the right on the main road through the village.*

THE PUB

The **Snooty Fox** is an excellent hostelry dating back to the 16th century. Flagstone floors, low beams and roaring log fires in winter or outside seating in summer make this a good place to be after a walk. The menu is extensive and includes a good range of sandwiches. Aberdeenshire steak cut to size is something of a speciality here and there is much to tempt the palate. Rich chocolate mousse cake with banana ice cream is one of its more 'wicked' offerings. Beers include Greene King, John Smith's and Guinness.

Food is served at lunchtime from 12 noon to 2 pm (2.30 pm on Sunday) and in the evening from 6.30 pm to 9.30 pm.
☎ *01832 733434*

1 Turn right out of the **Snooty Fox**, left down **Drayton Road** and almost immediately right into **Mill Lane**. Beyond the houses, the countryside opens up to you, giving lovely views across towards the parkland of the Drayton Estate. Red kites are often seen wheeling around in the sky here. Cross over a cattle grid and just before the second, climb the stile to the right into a large field and keep left along the fence, passing the back of a stone building. Where you meet an electric fence, go left into the corner and find a stile leading into the field ahead. Cross the next stile beside a metal gate and continue in the direction of

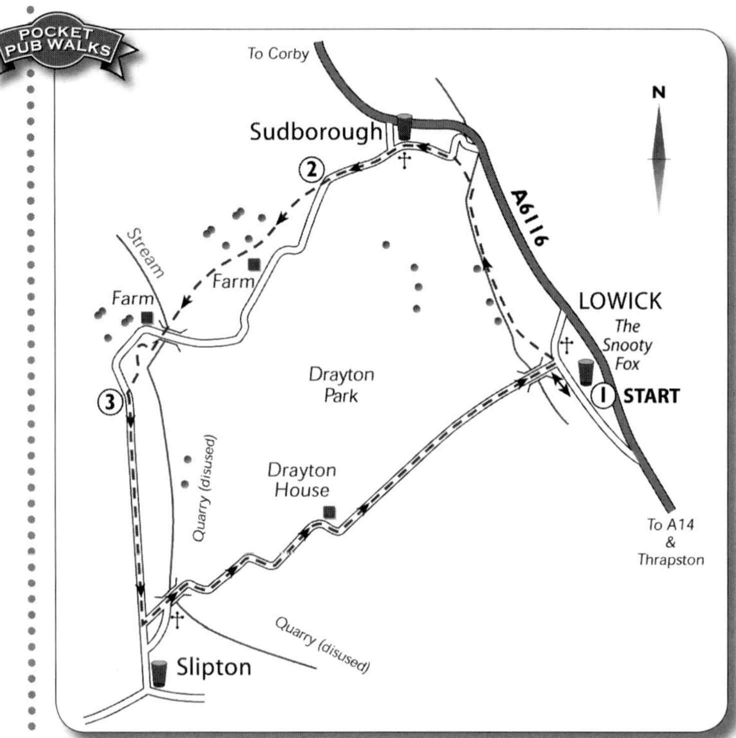

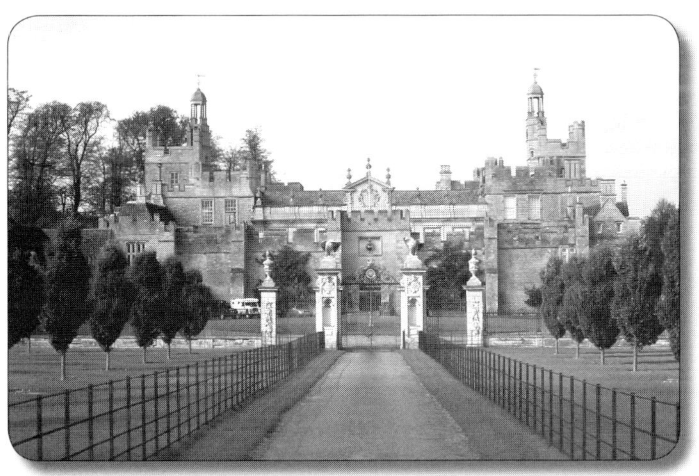

Drayton Hall stands in beautiful parkland.

the waymarkers. After passing through a rather ramshackle yard with its assortment of chickens, geese and guinea fowl, join the road ahead through the pretty village of **Sudborough**. The **Old Rectory** on the left has a very interesting and beautiful garden, which is often open under the National Gardens Scheme. The attractive **Vane Arms** is on the right. Walk through the village, crossing a bridge, and continue up the hill to where the road swings left.

2 Here, take the signed footpath to the right leading to the brow of the hill towards the telegraph poles on the horizon. Climb the stile and head right for a wooden gate by the spinney. In the hedge adjacent to this is another stile, which you climb, going into the next field. Waymarkers are in short supply from here but, never fear, the various instructions will keep you on track. Keeping the woodland on your right, follow round the field to a gap in the hedge and then down to another gap in the hedge, bottom left. Turn right towards a farm and follow the grass

verge as it curves round to meet the road. Turn right and on the far side of the tree in front, climb the stile with very great care! If you didn't get your feet wet this time, the waymarker leading straight ahead to a stile in the hedge opposite gives a second chance. To avoid this fate in the bog, go around the trees in the centre to circumnavigate the source of the spring. Go over the stile and proceed to a large single oak in the hedge opposite, emerging onto the road to **Slipton**.

3 Turn left along this quiet hedge-lined road with the deep disused quarries on either side and in about ½ mile reach yet another of Northamptonshire's pretty villages – **Slipton** – with its stone thatched cottages. Turn left at the sign to the church. Here you enter the **Drayton Estate** with its 'Private' notices (but this applies to vehicles not walkers). Follow the road up and round in front of the red-brick farm on the brow of the hill then turn left in front of a row of cottages and meet with a STOP sign on the gate. Ignore this and continue down the gravelly drive to **Drayton House**. Stay on the road, which leads round and in front of this gem. When you have finished admiring it, continue on the road through this lovely landscape back to **Drayton Road** and thence the **Snooty Fox**.

Place of interest nearby

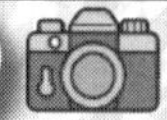

The fascinating **Lyveden New Bield**, off the A6116 going north towards Corby, is an unfinished building full of religious symbols and inscriptions set in the midst of moated terraced gardens, which are undergoing painstaking restoration by the National Trust.

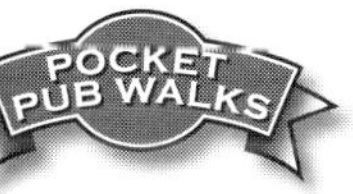

6 Rushton

The Thornhill Arms

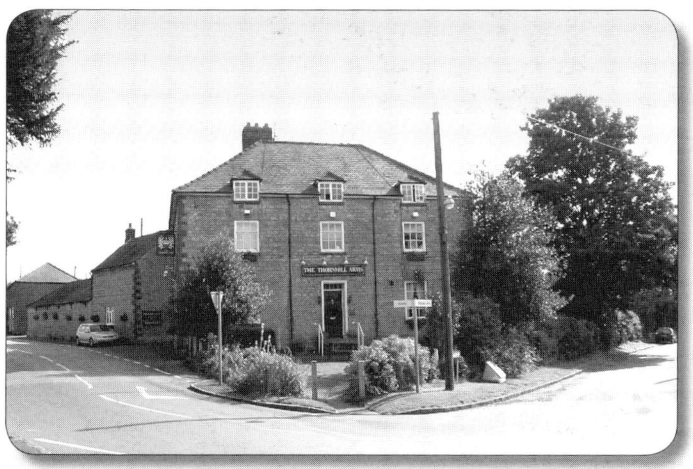

The village of Rushton, though only small, is home to the large and imposing Rushton Hall (now an hotel), which was owned by the Tresham family of Gunpowder Plot infamy. It was here, among other places, that Francis Tresham met with fellow conspirators to hatch the dastardly deed! Now all is peaceful, the only conflict being games of cricket in the charming ground below the church.

This walk takes you through gently undulating countryside with beautiful expansive views opening up. It visits the tiny village of Pipewell, once such a thriving place, and returns to Rushton via the intriguing Triangular Lodge.

Distance – 4½ miles.

OS Explorer 224 Corby, Kettering & Wellingborough. GR 842829.

Starting point The Thornhill Arms, which has a large car park for patrons. Otherwise, park in the road beside the pub.

How to get there *Rushton lies to the west of the Kettering to Corby road, the A6003. Approaching from Kettering, at the roundabout with the A43 continue straight ahead on Rockingham Road. Almost immediately turn left, signed to Glendon. Continue along this road until a sign to Rushton takes you right and then go right again into the village. The Thornhill Arms will be directly in front of you.*

THE PUB

The 300-year-old **Thornhill Arms** stands in an imposing position facing the church. It offers not only good food but accommodation too. The inside is spacious with oak beams and an inglenook fireplace adorned with horse brasses. In summer it is very pleasant to sit at tables in the garden and admire the view. The menu is extensive and appetising, offering 'Lite Bites' from soup to breaded whitebait and specials such as Caribbean coconut chicken or steak braised in red wine sauce. Sandwiches and jacket potatoes come with a multitude of fillings. The drinks on offer include Greene King IPA and Abbot Ale, John Smith's, Guinness and Strongbow cider.

Food is served at lunchtime from 12 noon to 2 pm and in the evening from 7 pm to 9.30 pm.
☎ *01536 710251*

1 Take the footpath and 'pocket park' sign on the other side of the road from the entrance to the pub car park. Going up the slight gradient, soon you will pass the entrance to the pocket park with its information board. A row of cottages appear on the right, followed shortly by a railway bridge.

2 Carry straight on along a wide grassy track with a tree-dotted hedge on the left. This is a good spot from which to enjoy the views that open up all around. Continue for about 1 mile before going downhill with the hedge now on the right. Ultimately head for a gabled cottage, near which the track is wide and overhung with trees (so it can be a bit muddy at times).

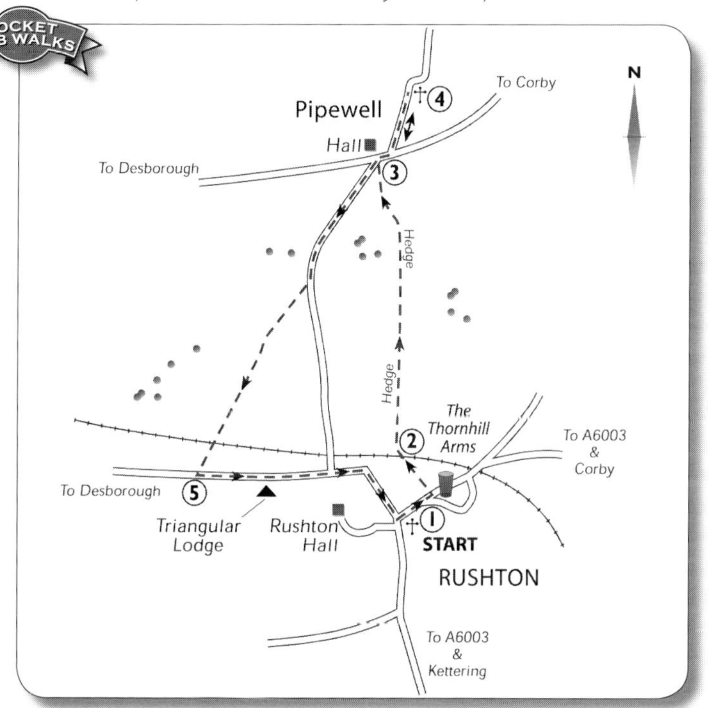

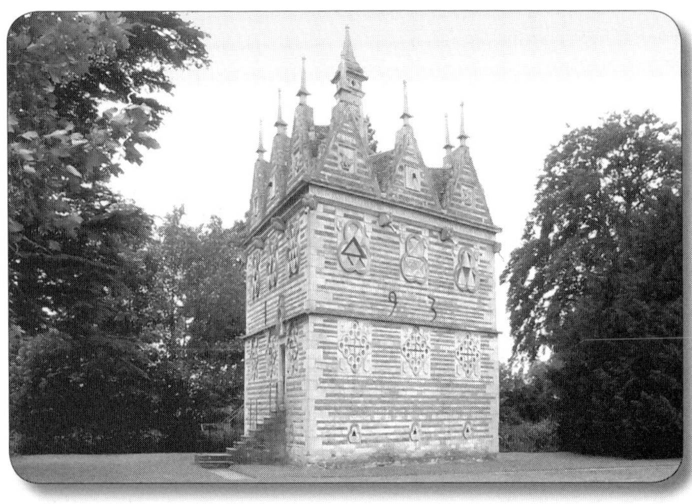

The fascinating triangular lodge.

3 After walking between fences, you emerge onto the **Corby/ Desborough road** opposite a Victorian 'gothic' lodge. Turn right, then left into the small village of **Pipewell**. Small it might be, but it was once the site of the largest and richest Cistercian abbey in southern England. It was here that Richard the Lionheart planned his third Crusade. Humps and hollows in the surrounding fields indicate the remains of the village.

4 Return to the Victorian lodge and take the road signposted to Kettering. After ½ mile, pass a lane marked 'unsuitable for heavy goods vehicles' and just before a farm, which you will see on the left, take a footpath signed right into a large field. Aim diagonally left for a gap in the woodland on the horizon. Continue straight ahead, keeping to the right-hand side of the hedge until you reach a gravel track. At this point continue diagonally right across a well marked path through a field

with the spire of **Desborough church** in the distance. Climb two stiles a few yards apart and, taking heed of the warning signs, cross the Midland mainline railway and carry on to the **Rushton/Desborough road**.

5 Turn left onto a fairly busy road. After some time a stone wall appears, behind which is the **Triangular Lodge** of Tresham fame. Step just inside the gate to read a brief history of the building. Continue on along the pavement beside the stone wall, which is rich ironstone, until you see a sign leading left into the village. Before turning, you may like to go on a little further to catch a glimpse of **Rushton Hall**, which is on the right. Return to the village, going through the churchyard to the **Thornhill Arms**.

Place of interest nearby

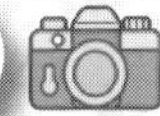

The **Triangular Lodge** (English Heritage) is one mile west of Rushton on the Desborough road. It is a unique and amazing building full of religious symbolism. Sir Thomas Tresham was languishing in gaol for his Catholic faith and whilst there designed the Lodge with all its references to the Trinity. Try and unravel the puns and puzzles on its walls!
☎ 01536 710761.

To the east of Rushton, south-east of Geddington, **Boughton House** is known as 'The English Versailles', although the house is a 500-year-old Tudor building and French additions were only added in the 16th century. It is owned by the Duke of Buccleuch and contains some wonderful treasures. The parkland is especially beautiful with woodland, lakes, riverside walks and avenues of historic trees. Children will enjoy the woodland play area when the weather is good.
☎ *01536 515731 for details of opening (the house itself is only open in August).*

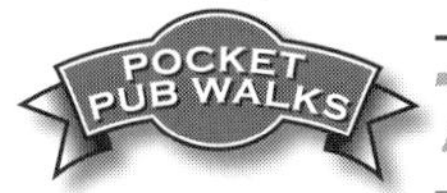

7 Little Harrowden

The Lamb Inn

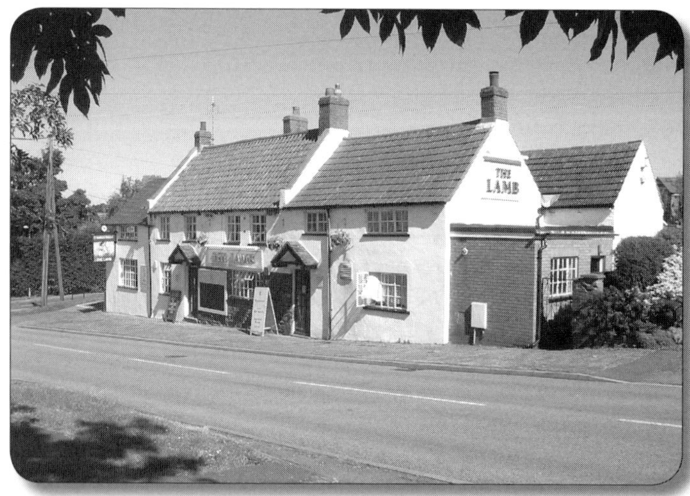

Little Harrowden is the longest and narrowest parish in Northamptonshire and has some interesting stone buildings. The 12th-century Norman church of St Mary the Virgin in the middle of the high street is a strange sight without either spire or tower! The spire fell down in 1703 and the west tower was demolished in the 19th century.

This is a delightful walk through fields in open countryside. It includes a visit to the charming village of Orlingbury with its large green shaded by mature trees and returns to Little Harrowden through pretty, undulating fields.

Distance – 4 miles

OS Explorer 224 Corby, Kettering & Wellingborough. GR 871716.

Starting point The Lamb Inn. Customers may leave their cars there while they walk – please seek permission of the landlord. Otherwise, park in the layby on the main road opposite the pub.

How to get there *The village is 5 miles south of Kettering. Turn off the A509 onto the B574 to Little Harrowden. The Lamb Inn is on the right-hand side on Orlingbury Road.*

THE PUB

The **Lamb Inn** is a cosy and welcoming pub with an oak beamed bar area and a sizeable restaurant. There are tables in the garden for use in clement weather. The building dates back to 1780 but the food is definitely 21st-century, interesting fare! There is a good selection of sandwiches and baguettes as well as light snacks. Chef specials are often available; otherwise dishes such as Thai chicken, succulent lamb or gammon with delicious desserts to follow will see you well satisfied. Wells Eagle and Bombardier, Hook Norton ale, Guinness or Foster's lager will slake your thirst.

Food is served Monday to Saturday from 12 noon to 2 pm and 7 pm to 9 pm; Sunday from 12 noon to 2.30 pm (no food is served Sunday evening).
☎ *01933 673300*

1 Turn left on leaving the pub, walking uphill to a roundabout. Turn right onto **Hardwick Road**. Continue along the verge and very shortly turn right through a kissing gate into a large

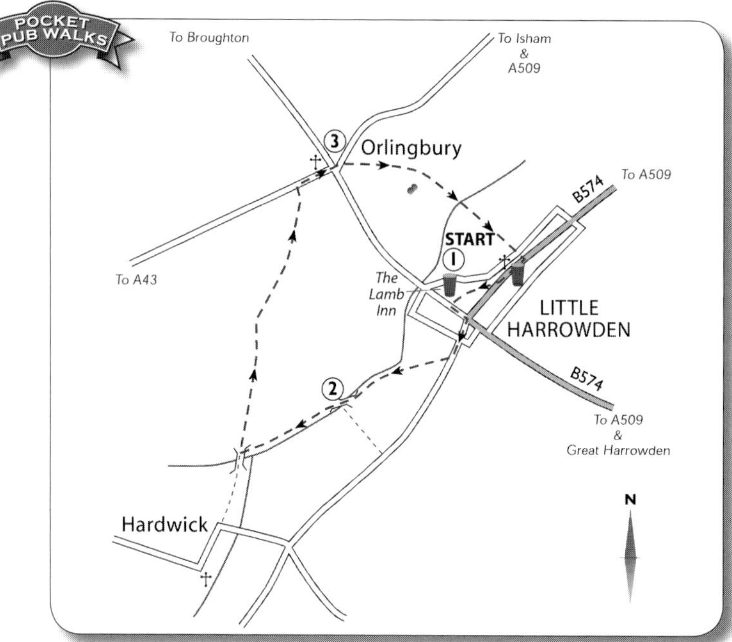

field. Follow the direction of the waymarker and where the path divides keep right down to a marker in a rather straggly hedge and then follow the hedge with the stream, which is a tributary of the River Ise, on the right.

2 The path crosses the stream and joins a byway, at which point walk right, keeping the hedge on the left, until you see a wooden bridge on the left. The path you want is on the right. Cross the large field diagonally right, aiming for the top of a pylon! At the gap in the hedge, go over a wooden plank and a sign to **Orlingbury** shows the way, aiming to the right of the church tower. Cross the stile and walk up the field, keeping the hedge on the right. At the top of the field turn

right over a double stile and continue diagonally left and over a stile beside a metal gate. Turn right over another stile and carry on, bearing left to a well signed gap in the hedge with a cattle trough. Proceed diagonally right across the field to yet another stile and go ahead to join the road, turning right into the village.

3 Pause awhile here on a bench on the green and savour the lovely surroundings. The **church of St Mary** was rebuilt in 1843, being paid for partly by the rector and partly by the then owner of Orlingbury Hall. It has a very beautiful contemporary stained-glass window erected in 1975 in memory of a villager who was a keen walker.

Go straight across the green – **Orlingbury Hall** is to the right – down **Rectory Lane** and **Dovecote Yard**, turning right just before **Lammas Close**, following the road through houses down a grassy track to a large field. Turn right, walking round the edge, keeping the hedge on the right until you reach a well-signed wooden bridge over a stream. Continue up the field to a kissing gate into a playing field, which you cross to another gate beside the school. Emerge onto the road where you turn right, passing in front of the little stone church with its missing spire. Just after **Pear Tree Close**, turn right, going downhill, to return to the **Lamb**.

Place of interest nearby

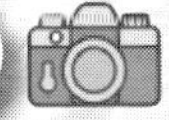

Sywell Aviation Museum, south-west of Little Harrowden and reached along Hardwick Road, is well worth a visit. Its aim is to preserve the history of aviation in Northamptonshire. Various events take place throughout the year at the aerodrome and you could always book a flying lesson!
☎ *01604 491112.*

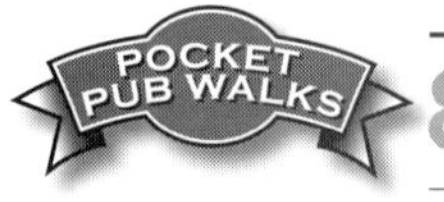

8 Lamport

The Swan

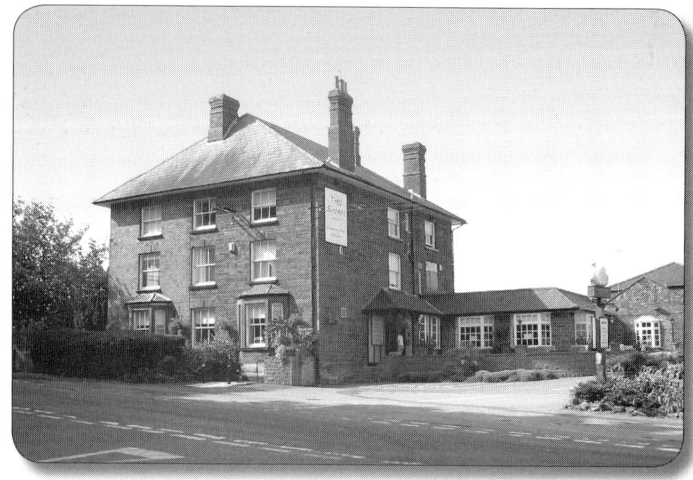

Lamport is a small village with a large mansion in its midst. Lamport Hall, built in the 15th century, has been the home of the Isham family since 1560. It now belongs to the Lamport Hall Trust and is used for corporate events but the hall and gardens can be visited sporadically from Easter to mid October. The lovely gardens were home to the original garden gnome!

This is a delightful walk in quiet countryside with beautiful views. The way passes through the village of Scaldwell before visiting the hamlet of Hanging Houghton and joining the Brampton Valley Way.

Distance – 4½ miles.

OS Explorer 223 Northampton & Market Harborough. GR 756746.

Starting point The Swan in Harborough Road. There is a large car park beside the pub for patrons. Otherwise, there is roadside parking in the village.

How to get there *Lamport is on the A508 Market Harborough/ Northampton road 8 miles south of Market Harborough.*

THE PUB

The **Swan** is an imposing pub on the main road, recently refurbished in the modern style, with a large garden and patio area giving wonderful views across the valley. The menu is extensive and mouth watering. The 'simple food' category includes soup and sandwiches with a variety of fillings, such as beef and mustard mayonnaise. Sea bass fillet and roast venison are among the more substantial dishes. The desserts sound very good! Beers include Young's, Wells Bombardier and Adnams.

Food is served Monday to Saturday from 12 noon to 3 pm and 6 pm to 9 pm; and on Sunday from 12 noon to 4 pm.
☎ *01604 686555*

1 On leaving the **Swan**, turn right onto the A508 and as you go you will be able to enjoy the lovely views across open countryside towards **Guilsborough** on the right and catch glimpses of **Lamport Hall** to the left. The imposing entrance to the hall with its twin pillars surmounted by two white swans comes into view, followed very quickly by a footpath sign leading left to **Scaldwell**. Follow the path through the trees until you reach the ruins of an old

stone barn (now just a very low wall). At this point, the village of Scaldwell can be seen across the fields to the right and it is to here that your path leads. Go diagonally across the field to a large gap in the hedge and continue ahead, keeping the hedge on your left. The correct path goes diagonally across the field but there is a wide grassy margin skirting the edge and sweeping round to the same waymarker, which will lead you to **Scaldwell**. After the third field you are directed to a path bisecting a garden and onto the road.

2 Turn right through this pretty village with its honey-coloured stone cottages and well tended gardens, ignoring signs to right and left, and after passing **Sundial House** and **The Grange**, turn

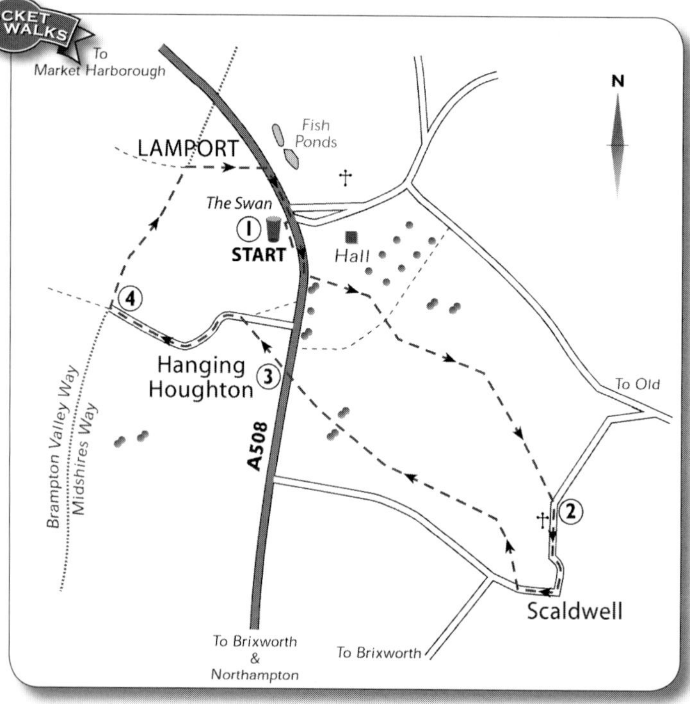

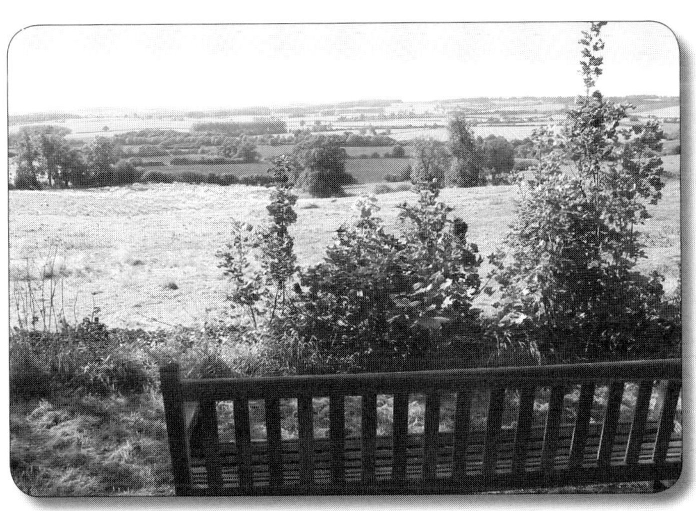

The glorious view across the valley.

right down **Peter`s Road**. Here a footpath sign on the left leads down alongside a clipped hedge and then several waymarkers show the route ahead. A waymarker in the corner of one field is a little misleading in that it appears to lead very sharp left but in fact you go through the hedge and carry on left, keeping the hedge on your left. Continue to a gap in the hedge where there is a waymark hidden behind a small sapling. Go straight across the field to enter a newly planted copse of oak, pine and birch. On emerging, go diagonally right to the far side of the field. The waymarker leading to the road is just beyond a maple tree in the hedge on the left.

3 Cross the road, turn right and follow the sign to **Hanging Houghton**, which goes diagonally across a single field, pointing to the first house and a stile. Keep right and join the road. At this point there is a choice of route; either follow the footpath

sign right from the centre of the village, taking you straight back to the A508 and thence to the pub, or continue left, walking down the road and swinging left, with beautiful views over the surrounding countryside, until you come to the **Houghton Crossing** on the **Brampton Valley Way**. This is a 14-mile linear park – be assured you are only doing a small part of it – linking Northampton and Market Harborough.

4 Here turn right, making use of the well placed seats along the route, which is lined with traditional hedgerows and ancient meadows. This is a car free path but watch out for the silent cyclist. After some distance, a large fingerpost shows the way, right, to **Lamport Hall** and **village**. On reaching the road, turn right to the **Swan**.

Place of interest nearby

All Saints' church at Brixworth 'is the most imposing architectural memorial of the seventh century surviving north of the Alps', according to Pevsner. Is there any more to say? From Lamport continue down the A508 towards Northampton and turn right at the first roundabout.

Brixworth Country Park at Pitsford Water, south of Lamport along the A508, is a lovely area with waymarked trails around the reservoir, grassy meadows and woodland. There is something for everyone to enjoy and the visitor centre is a delight. There is also an excellent café, which can get very busy at weekends in summer. For the fit, there are bicycles for hire or you could arrange fly-fishing or sailing tuition!
☎ *01604 883920.*

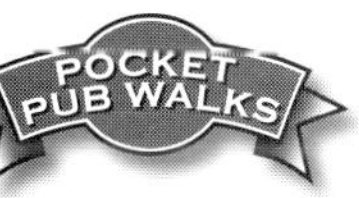

9 Yardley Hastings

The Rose and Crown

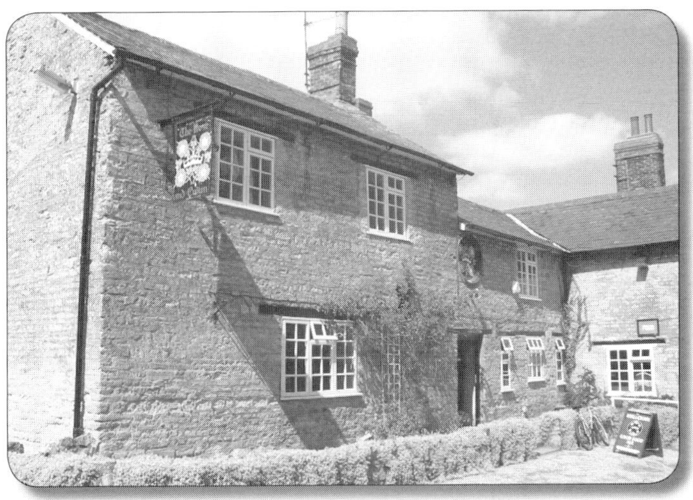

Yardley Hastings is a moderately large village with stone cottages and pretty gardens. The church of St Andrew contains an unusual memorial to Edward Lye who inspired Dr Johnson; it is adorned with a carved ink well, quill and dictionary. Castle Ashby, the village's near neighbour, is an outstanding estate village with a magnificent mansion in its midst.

This walk takes you from Yardley Hastings into the beautiful pastures of the Castle Ashby Estate, much of it designed by Capability Brown. One can stand and admire the mansion at close quarters through the magnificent gates. The route back is through lush meadows bordering the brook. In autumn the hedgerows along here are laden with blackberries.

Distance – 4½ miles.

OS Explorer 207 Newport Pagnell & Northampton South. GR 863568.

Starting point The Rose and Crown where patrons can leave their cars in the large car park while they walk – please seek permission. Otherwise there is parking on the road near to the pub.

How to get there *Yardley Hastings is 7 miles east of Northampton, just north of the A428. Take the first turn signed into Yardley Hastings and follow the road through the village. At the fork, turn left and the pub is on the right.*

THE PUB

The **Rose and Crown** is a cosy pub, probably built in the fifteen hundreds. Its bar is oak beamed with stone flagged floors. The seating area is very pleasant and in addition one can sit outside on fine days and children can enjoy the play equipment. The food on offer is varied and good. There are sandwiches, jacket potatoes and baguettes with a multitude of fillings as well as delicious hickory chicken, steak pie and a carvery every day. Beers include John Smith's and different ales each week, also Foster's and Kronenbourg lagers.

Food is served at lunchtime (Tuesday to Sunday) from 12 noon to 2 pm; in the evening it is available from 6 pm to 9 pm on Tuesday to Saturday and from 7 pm to 9 pm on Sunday. The pub is closed on Monday.

☎ *01604 696276*

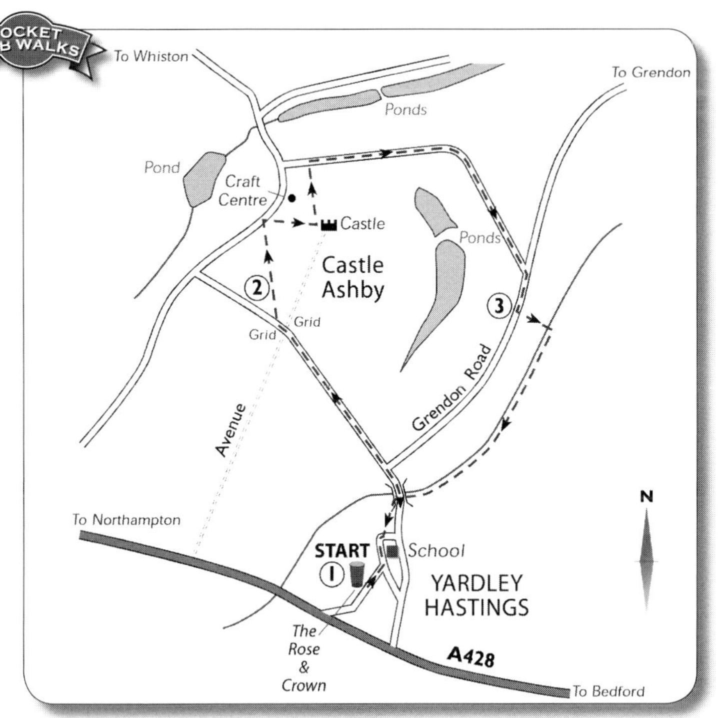

1 Turn left out of the **Rose and Crown**, passing a converted chapel, which is now a National Resource Centre, and keep bearing left down **Castle Ashby Road**. At a little grass triangle, veer left into **Little Lane**, which runs between a brook and a charming row of stone cottages. On reaching a bridge, cross it and enter a wooded area, keeping the brook on the left until the next bridge where you turn left onto the road to **Castle Ashby**. Go over the cattle grid and carry on, admiring the imposing avenue, which leads to the magnificent **Castle Ashby House**. The drive in its entirety runs for 3½ miles. The house is owned by the Compton

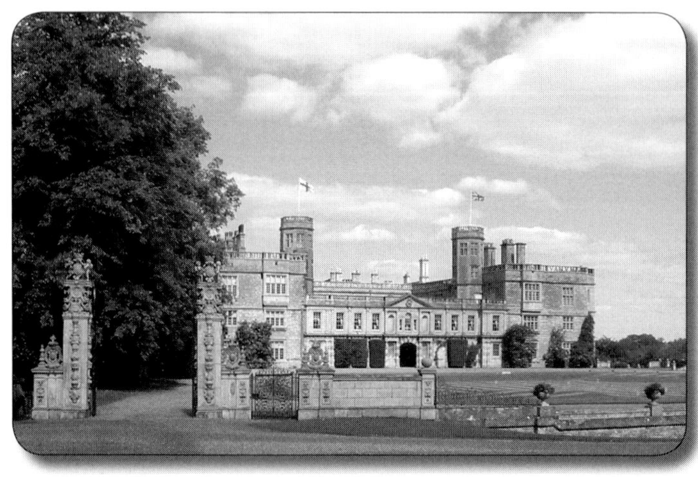

Castle Ashby House.

family, who bought 'a ruined castle' in the 1530s. The church of St Mary Magdalene lies within the garden.

2 Having crossed the second grid, take the footpath right, signed diagonally across the field to a waymarker and stile. Take a line left of the lone oak to a metal gate at the road. Turn immediately right into a wooded area, which soon gives a good view of the magnificent gates of the house. For the Latin scholar, the openwork inscriptions on the parapet are from Psalms 127 and 128. A this point you could turn right in front of them to visit the gardens, open 10 am to 4.30 pm, before carrying on with the walk, which goes left onto a path in front of a house and past a car park. Carry on straight ahead (resisting, if you can, the temptation of a visit to the **Rural Shopping Yard**) until reaching the tiny village green before the pretty **Falcon pub**, with its two chestnut trees. Turn right down the road and through a metal gate. The narrow road goes through an idyllic pastoral scene

where sheep graze among the beautiful trees, with glimpses of the **Grendon lakes**, which are generally ringed with anglers, to the left and views of the house and its lakes to the right.

3 On reaching the T-junction, turn right, signed to **Yardley Hastings**. In about 200 yards, turn left down a bridleway to a concrete bridge, which you cross. Then go right, following an obvious path through lush grassland and over grassy mounds beside the brook, which runs in an ever-deepening gully. On reaching the bridge at **Yardley Hastings**, cross the road and retrace your steps to the **Rose and Crown**.

Place of interest nearby

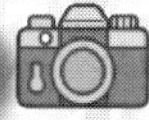

All Saints' at Earls Barton is one of the finest Saxon pre-Conquest churches in England and can be seen for miles around, including at night when it is floodlit. The tower is particularly interesting and overlooks a Norman castle motte. From Yardley Hastings, take the road signed to Castle Ashby and thence to Earls Barton on the other side of the A45.

The village of **Castle Ashby** is full of interest. You may walk in the gardens of **Castle Ashby House**, for a small fee, but the house itself is not open to the public. Beautiful parkland with lakes and pastures dotted with sheep makes this an idyllic place.
☎ *01604 696232.*

The **Rural Shopping Yard** at Castle Ashby has some unusual shops (the delicatessen is particularly mouth watering) as well as a coffee shop serving light lunches. Closed on Monday (except bank holidays).
☎ *01604 696232.*

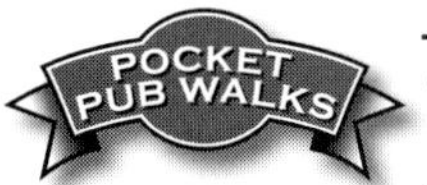

10 Little Bringston

The Saracen's Head

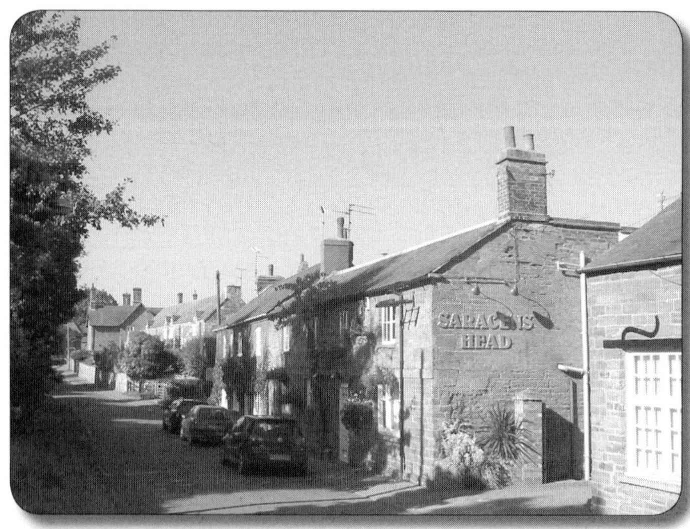

The hamlet of Little Brington has its place in history for, among other things, being the one-time home of the two grandsons of Lawrence Washington of Sulgrave whose descendent was George Washington. St John's church on the outskirts of the village is a strange sight with only the tower and spire sitting forlornly in a tiny churchyard. The building fell into disrepair and was due for demolition but was saved by the intervention of the RAF as it was on their maps and used as a landmark by the pilots!

Little Brington

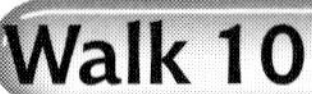

This is an interesting walk through field and meadow with a visit to Great Brington and the Althorp Estate along with the chance to view the Spencer Chapel in the church.

Distance – 4 miles.

OS Explorer 223 Northampton & Market Harborough. GR 663637.

Starting point The Saracen's Head. Customers may leave their cars in the car park while they walk – please ask first. There is also space to park on the roadside near the pub.

How to get there Little Brington is approx 5½ miles west of Northampton and east of Daventry, lying between Flore and Great Brington. The Saracen's Head is on Main Street and is recognisable with an apple tree on the front growing from the foundations!

THE PUB

The **Saracen's Head** is a charming 16th-century pub of dark stone. The cosy interior with its fireplace gives way to modern extensions and a large and attractive gravelled area with tables and umbrellas. Baguettes and tortilla wraps with delicious fillings are on offer as well as light bites and soup. There are main dishes to suit all tastes, among them beef and Guinness pie, chargrilled haloumi kebabs and chicken or vegetable curry – to name but a few. Beers include Timothy Taylor's Landlord, Greene King IPA, John Smith's and a guest ale along with Guinness, Foster's lager and Strongbow cider on draught.

Food is served from 12 noon to 2 pm and 6 pm to 9.30 pm on Monday to Saturday and 12 noon to 7 pm on Sunday.
☎ *01604 770640*

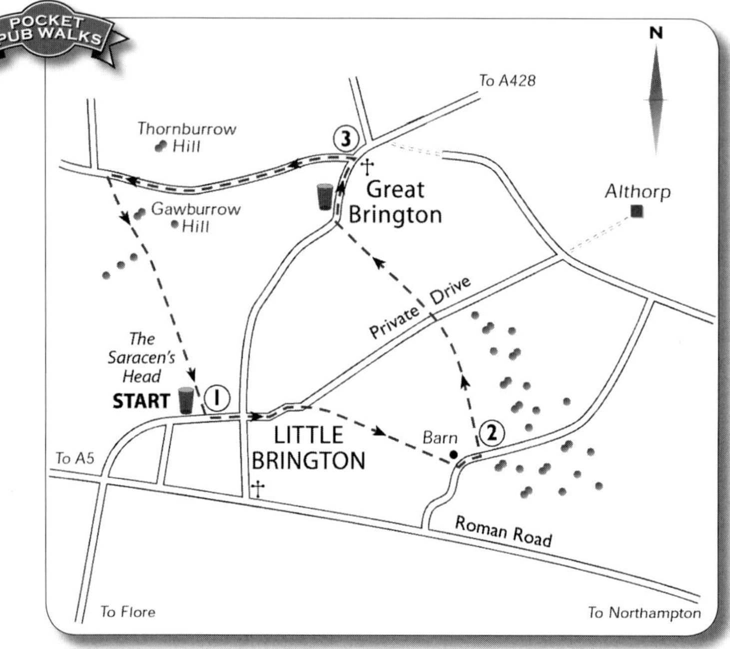

1 On leaving the **Saracen's Head**, turn left along the road. At the road junction and just before crossing over to a wooden gate on the drive to **Althorp House**, take a few paces to the right to see **Washington House** with its inscription above the door and a stone sundial with the Washington arms nearby. After the second gate take the footpath right, across a large field. The line you want is rather more to the right than the sign would indicate, the waymarker being about 50 yards to the left of a large ash tree and hidden in the hedge. From here follow the markers ultimately towards a red brick barn and right to the road where you turn left.

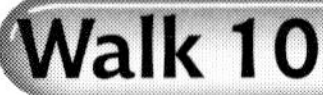

2 Fifty yards on, a footpath sign indicates the route to **Great Brington**. Cross the large field directly to the waymarker, taking you once again over the drive to the house and thence to the village. On reaching the road, turn right up the hill, passing the attractive **Fox and Hounds pub**. A **Macmillan Way** marker leads up to the **church of St Mary** with its commanding views over the countryside.

3 Cross the road from the church and take the single track road towards **Whilton**. On either side are tree-topped humps that could be burial mounds; to the right **Thornburrow Hill** and to the left **Gawburrow**. Continue for some distance, ignoring the many footpath signs, until just before a roughly surfaced track to the right, take the footpath signed left up the hill. At the top of the field go through the gate and head for a gate at the end of a line of trees. Squeeze through the gap and turn right up to a stile. From here, follow the markers, with the spire of **Little Brington church** in your sights. Ultimately climb the stile beside a tin-roofed hut to reach the road. Turn right for the **Saracen's Head**.

Place of interest nearby

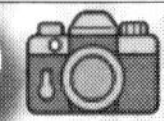

Coton Manor, to the north of the A428, is surrounded by a simply beautiful garden; it is a must for the horticulturally inclined! A visit in spring to the five acre wood full of bluebells is a sight to behold. The manor is not open to the public but light meals are available in a charming courtyard. There is a small shop and plants are on sale.

☎ *01604 740219 for opening times*

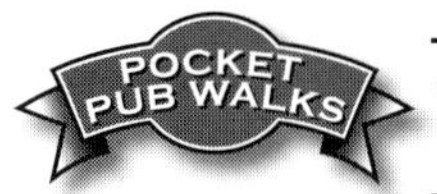

11 Welton

The White Horse

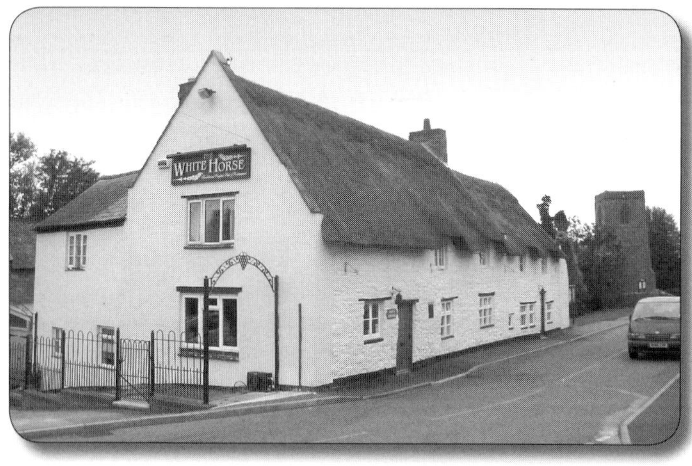

The charming village of Welton sits on a limestone hill near the Warwickshire border, its name being derived from the many wells and springs in the area. To the south there is a beautiful stretch of water surrounded by cedars, among other trees, which have preservation orders on them. This is an ornamental lake once attached to Welton Place.

This delightful walk passes the village of Ashby St Ledgers with its association with the Gunpowder Plot and on through the pleasant meadows to join the towpath of the Grand Union Canal before returning across the fields to Welton.

Distance – 5½ miles.

OS Explorer 222 Rugby & Daventry. GR 581661.

Starting point The White Horse at Welton. Patrons may leave their cars in the pub car park while they are walking, but please ask first. There is also roadside parking in the village.

How to get there *Welton is 2 miles north of Daventry and east of the A361. To get to the pub, turn right off the A361 two miles north of Daventry(to Welton, on Ashby Road). Turn right into the village down Well Lane, right at the T-junction and you will see the pub on the left.*

THE PUB

The **White Horse** is a welcoming inn with a small low-beamed bar area and restaurant. The garden is sizeable as is the patio area. Good plain food is served and includes a selection of sandwiches, paninis and snacks. For the more hungry, steak and ale pie or liver and bacon are but two of the home-made dishes. Roasts are served on Sundays. The dessert menu changes from day to day. Jennings Bitter, St Austell Tinners and Greene King Abbot Ale are just some of the beers on offer.

Food is served at lunchtime from 12 noon to 2 pm on Monday to Friday and 12 noon to 3 pm on Sunday; it is available every evening from 6.30 pm to 9.30 pm.
☎ *01327 702820*

1 Turn right out of the **White Horse** up to the junction and go left. Just beyond the post box turn right at the sign leading between the houses and carry on up the field beside the

hedge. Some 50 yards before the metal gate at the top go right through the hedge across a wooden plank into the field and head diagonally left to the hedge. Keeping this on your left, proceed along the wide grassy verge for some distance and climb the stile onto the road. Follow the road sign to **Ashby St Ledgers**. Turn right at the junction to the most historic part of the village. Here is the interesting **church of St Leodegarius** (corrupted to Ledgers) with its medieval wall paintings and three-tier pulpit. Beside the church is the manor house once owned by the Catesby family of Gunpowder Plot infamy. Much of the planning took place here and it was to this place that the conspirators returned, following the failure, before fleeing to Staffordshire, where Catesby and Percy were shot. Before

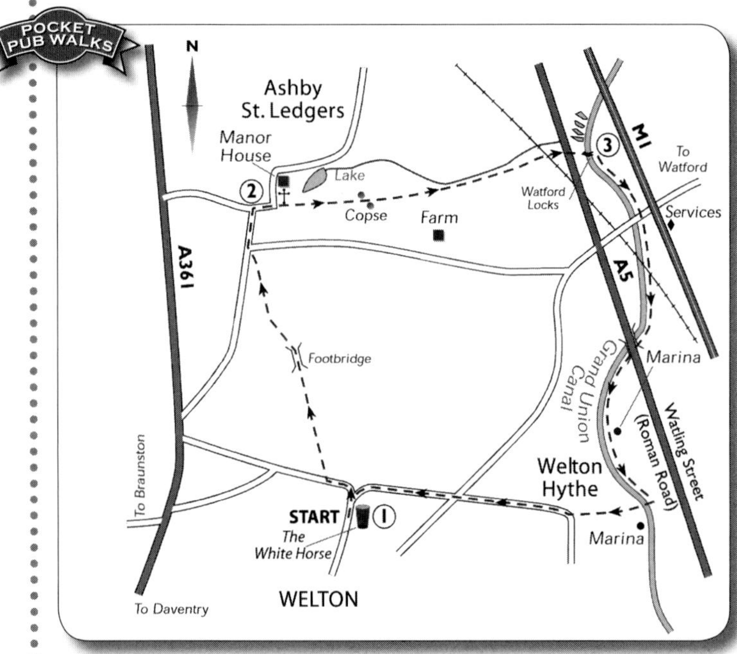

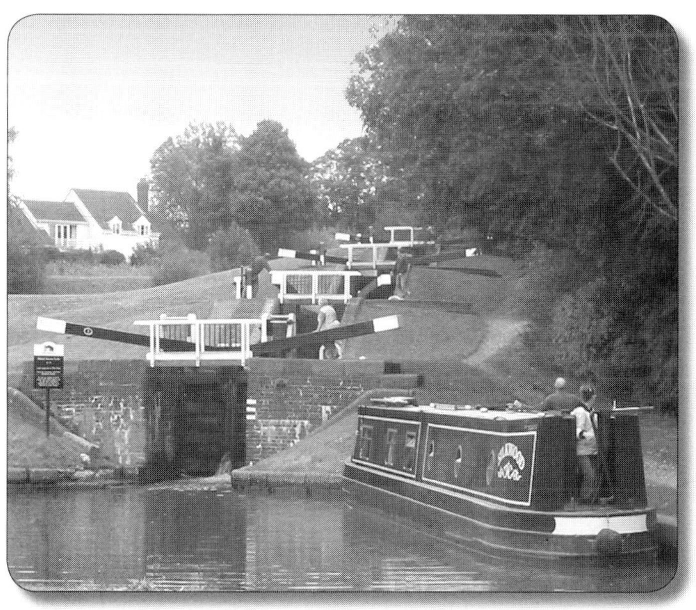

The flight of locks at Watford.

continuing with the walk, you may like to wander around the village to see the Lutyens thatched cottages in the main street along with some other attractive houses.

2 Take the footpath down beside the churchyard and proceed up the hill to a lone stile and ahead to the hedge. Do not go straight on as the next sign might indicate, but walk diagonally left down to a small copse, which you enter via a well hidden stile in the hedge. Continue through the copse and over a stile into the field. Ignore the large footpath sign, which would go straight ahead, and walk diagonally left to the hedge alongside the brook. Carry on until the waymarkers guide you under the railway line to the A5. Cross the road, turning left to a sign

taking you up to **Watford Locks**. There are seven locks, which lift the water over 50 ft. Forty-five minutes of hard labour could see one through!

3 Cross the canal to the towpath and turn right, enjoying the sight of so many boats using this **Leicester Arm** of the **Grand Union Canal** and navigating the locks. The sound of traffic is soon left behind, enabling you to enjoy this lovely walk of about 2 miles along the towpath. Go under the bridge just before **Welton Hythe Marina** then immediately left up to the road. Cross the bridge and a waymarker will lead left and then right through a gate alongside a private conservatory. Veer left and, keeping the hedge on your right, head up and round the field. Finally pass through a gate onto the road and continue ahead to the crossroads. Here go straight ahead for about ¼ mile to return to **Welton**. At the little green, go ahead, signed to **Daventry**, and return to the **White Horse**.

Place of interest nearby

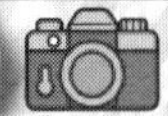

Braunston – reached to the west of Welton, across the A361 – lies at the junction of the Grand Union and Oxford canals and has the busiest flight of locks in the country. The village itself is situated on a hill above the canal; it has two pubs as well as a few shops, but most activity centres on the canal and marina. Stroll along the towpath, where you will see the Stop House at which tolls were collected from passing boats. There is a shop near the bottom lock selling food and ice creams as well as souvenirs..

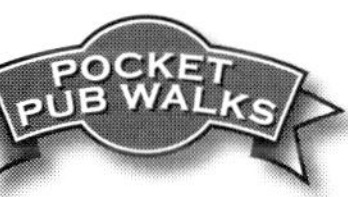

12 Stoke Bruerne

The Navigation

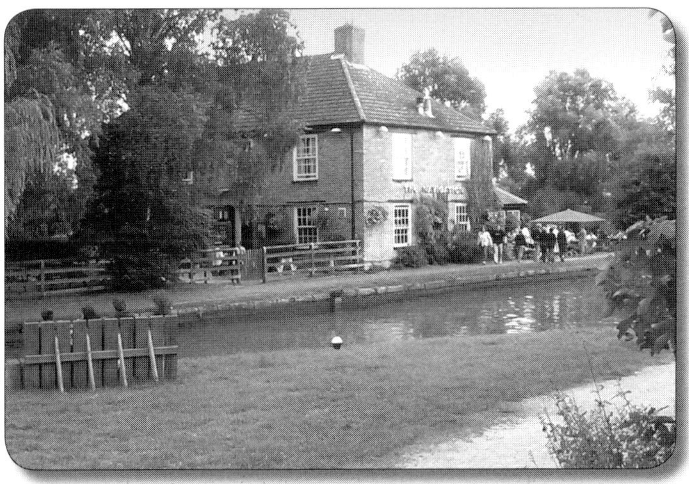

Stoke Bruerne is an interesting village not just because of the Grand Union Canal, which bisects it; it was mentioned in the Domesday Book and has long had its place in history. The canal, of course, has brought great hustle and bustle to its centre, with barges navigating the locks, and the wharves busy in summer with people visiting the excellent museum or the Boat Inn. In the past, coal and other commodities went by barge from Birmingham to London; the accent today is on leisure rather than commerce.

The walk takes you above the Blisworth Tunnel along a delightfully shaded lane, thence through meadows and alongside a wandering brook. It returns over the sheep-dotted pastures of the Stoke Park Pavilions.

Distance – 3½ miles.

OS Explorer 207 Newport Pagnell & Northampton South. GR 745498.

Starting point The Navigation pub beside the canal has a large car park to its rear. There is also a pay and display parking area behind the museum.

How to get there *Stoke Bruerne is 4 miles east of Towcester and 7 miles south of Northampton. The village is well signed off the A508. To reach the pub, continue through the village but bear left before the bridge and it is on the right.*

THE PUB The large **Navigation** is right beside the canal, giving good views of the canal traffic, more especially so if you sit outside in the garden to watch the colourful barges glide by. Foodwise there is just about everything one could want: mini grills, sandwiches, baguettes and jacket potatoes, along with steak and ale pie, chargrilled sirloin, fresh salmon and many other dishes. The dessert menu looks very tempting too! Jennings Cumberland Ale and Sneck Lifter, Foster's, Carlsberg, Guinness and Strongbow cider are all on offer from the bar.

Food is served from 12 noon to 9 pm every day.
☎ 01604 864988

1 From the car park behind the **Navigation**, take the steps by the disabled parking area onto the towpath and turn right towards the bridge. Cross the road, going ahead to enjoy the busy scene

at the lockside with boats being guided into the lock, some more expertly than others! Continue along, passing the museum, towards the mouth of the **Blisworth Tunnel**. This amazing feat of engineering was finally opened in 1805 after a previous tunnel collapsed and is the ninth longest canal tunnel in the world, being 3,076 yards long. The path goes up the slope, but before taking it, it might be of interest to approach the tunnel to read some more interesting information about its construction. Continue for a short time and on the left is a wooden sign just short of a farm track. Turn left here.

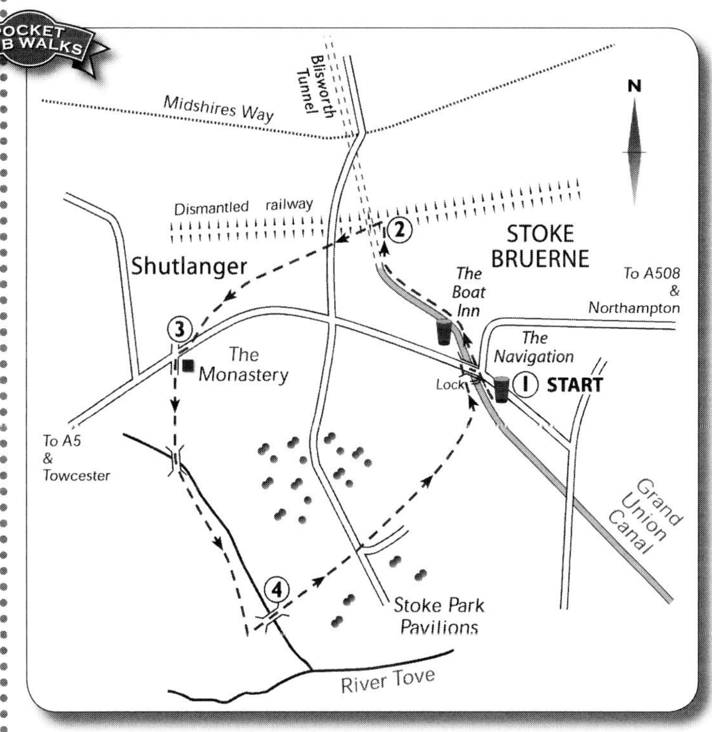

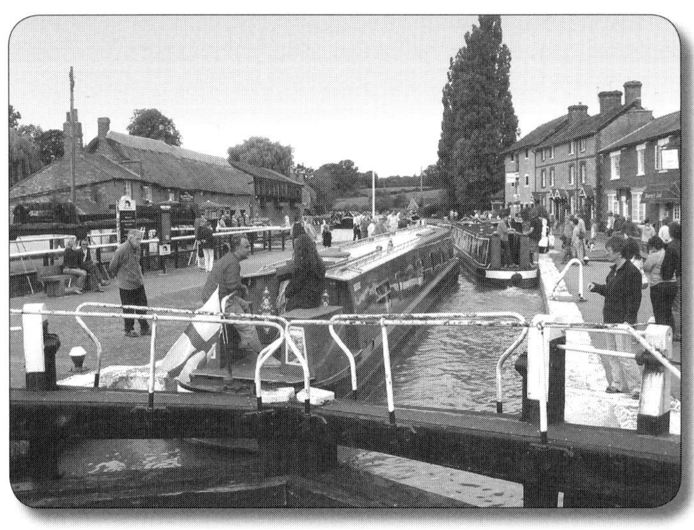

A busy scene along the Grand Union Canal at Stoke Bruerne.

2 The short grassy path leads onto the aforesaid track, which you follow to a metal barn and thence a road. Cross and go down a long track to the bottom of the field. Bear left uphill with the hedge on the left. Cross two fields and go through a metal gate onto a road.

3 Turn right to the crossroads at **Shutlanger** and left down **Water Lane**. On the left is an area designated '**The Monastery'** though this is no longer in evidence. Keep on ahead down a bridleway, ignoring signs to left and right. Here the countryside opens out and you cross the field, aiming left of the farm on the hill, to a wooden bridge with a gate. Cross this and turn left to follow the brook, which meanders along for a considerable distance. It eventually turns away to the left, leaving you to continue ahead by the ditch. The hedgerows here are rich in sloes and wild apples in the autumn but don't be tempted – both are very bitter!

4 When you arrive at a bewildering array of gates, follow the waymarker sharp left over a stile beside a metal gate. Carry on up the field, going to the top left corner to a gate onto the drive of **Stoke Park Pavilions**, which are to the right. Having crossed the road, go straight ahead through a metal gate and follow the marker to a line of poplars – once the driveway to the Pavilions. Go through a gate and turn left along a hedge-lined grassy track abundant with wildlife before passing a pocket park to arrive back at the village.

Place of interest nearby

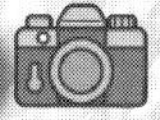

Look no further than the wonderful **Waterways Museum** housed in an old three-storey corn mill on the wharf beside the canal. It is a treasure house of artefacts with working models depicting and portraying all aspects of life on the water. The shop sells souvenirs as well as painted canalware and there is a little café.
☎ *01604 862229.*

Stoke Park Pavilions, reached from the Shutlanger road out of Stoke Bruerne and open daily in August, were begun in about 1640 by Inigo Jones but completed by another architect after the interruption of the Civil War. The Pavilions still stand but the house itself was destroyed by a fire in 1886. The beautiful gardens are undergoing restoration.
☎ *01604 862329.*

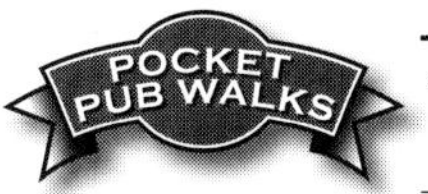

13 Charwelton

The Fox and Hounds

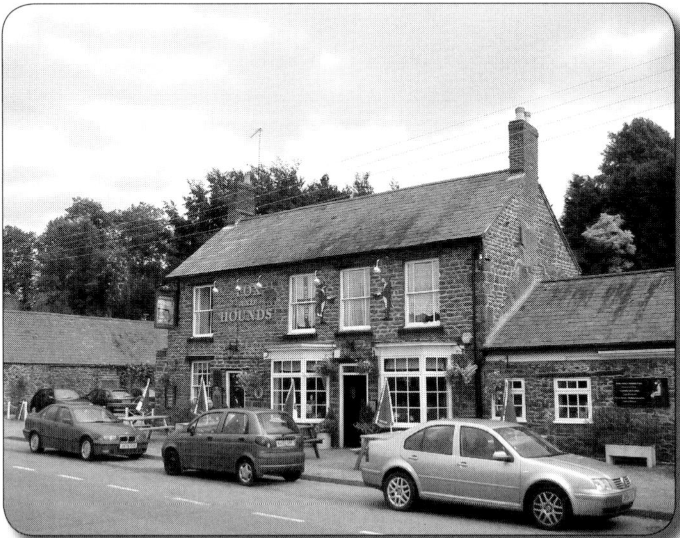

The delightful little packhorse bridge that lies alongside the main road is rarely noticed by the motorist bowling along the busy A361 through this small village. It is only three feet wide but is reckoned to be one of the finest in the country. Not far away, just over the meadows, lies the tiny enclave of Church Charwelton where Holy Trinity church stands in the midst of a deserted medieval village with its still-evident fishponds. The church contains many treasures, among them some excellent brasses that are now underneath a length of carpet, which you are at liberty to roll up! A magnificent tomb-chest of the Andrewes family who lived at Manor Farm next to the church in the 15th century was removed briefly in 2002 to Tate Britain as part of an exhibition of medieval treasures. The key can be obtained from the farm.

This is a delightful walk by streams and through large meadows. Beyond Church Charwelton, beautiful views of Badby Downs soon open up before you visit what was the Royal Manor of Fawsley where Elizabeth I really did sleep! The little church of St Mary lies snugly below the hall, set in lovely parkland. It is then an idyllic walk back to Charwelton.

Distance – 5 miles.

OS Explorer 206 Edgehill & Fenny Compton. GR 534561.

Starting point The Fox and Hounds where customers may leave their cars while they walk, but please seek permission. There is also some parking on the side turning south of the pub.

How to get there *The Fox and Hounds at Charwelton is 4 miles south of Daventry on the A361.*

THE PUB The **Fox and Hounds** is a deceptively large public house and restaurant built in the 17th century, with a 20th-century conservatory giving onto a small seating area outside. The menu is extensive, with portions to match for the hungry walker. The dessert menu, which changes regularly, looked very tempting when we were there – but there was just no room! Hook Norton ales, Guinness and Carling, Foster's, Stella and Grolsch lagers are among the beers available.

Food is served at lunchtime from 12 noon to 2 pm on Monday to Friday and from 12 noon to 3.30 pm at weekends; in the evening it is available from 6 pm to 9.30 pm throughout the week.
☎ *01327 262358*

1 Turn right out of the **Fox and Hounds**, crossing the packhorse bridge and turning right at the war memorial onto the **Jurassic Way**. Follow the markers to the road. Turn left and then right into a field, enjoying the sight of various wildfowl and maybe the odd heron alongside the old fishponds, continuing until you arrive at the isolated **church of Holy Trinity** with its reddish

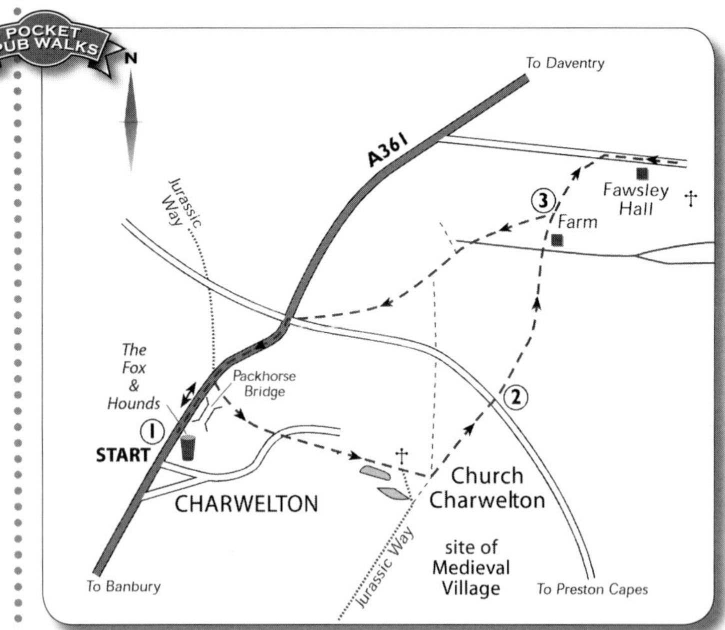

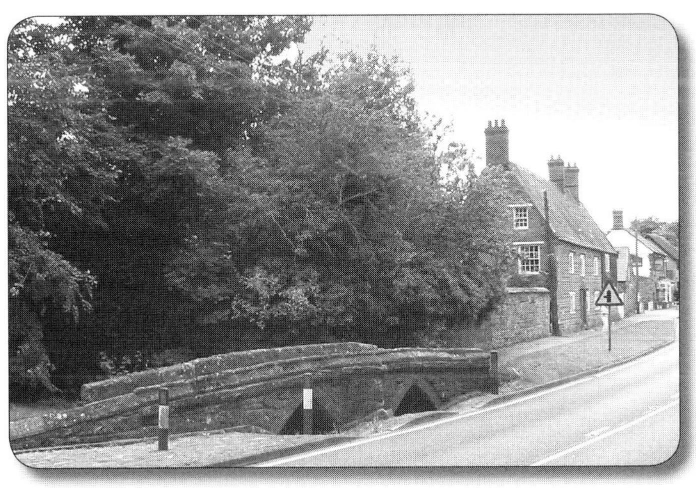

The packhorse bridge in Charwelton.

stone spotted with lichen. On leaving the church, bear left to the corner of a wire fenced enclosure, following it up and round to the right to a metal gate with a track in front of it leading to the road.

2 Cross the road and go through two metal gates to the top of the hill, enjoying the lovely sight of the **Badby Downs** before you. Carry on with the wire fencing on the right and go ahead through a metal gate onto a track leading to **Fawsley Farm**. A waymarker leads you up the hill past **The Granary** with its 'Boutique Conferencing and Accommodation'. Soon after this you will see a metal gate on the left with a marker, to which you will return after visiting **Fawsley Hall** and the church. To do this, continue up the road, turning right past a large stone building, admiring the beautiful pastoral scene that opens up on the left. Fawsley Hall, now a hotel, began life in the 15th century in the ownership of the Knightley family. In more recent times a kindly

Lady Knightley gave sanctuary to John Merrick, otherwise known as 'The Elephant Man', to shield him from the relentless gaze of the public.

3 Having retraced your steps, now follow the waymarker down to the brook, walking alongside it to a point where you cross it near a small pond. Go ahead with the hedge on your left (not up the hill) and where it joins another across the bottom of the field look carefully for two wooden gates, one behind another, with a marker on the far side. Follow the diverted footpath up and round to the left. Turn right at the gate and go ahead to a hedge. Keeping this on the right, continue down to a gap with a marker directing you across a large field to the far left corner – but if this is muddy, carry on to the road and turn right. At the junction, take the **Charwelton** road along the verge to the pub.

Place of interest nearby

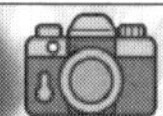

Canons Ashby – reached via the A361 to the south of Charwelton, turning off to Eydon – is an Elizabethan manor house owned by the National Trust but once the home of the Dryden family. It contains some interesting wall paintings and in fact little has changed since 1710. The gardens are a delight with beautiful herbaceous borders and the orchard is stocked with 16th-century varieties of fruit. The little tearoom serves light lunches and teas.
☎ *01327 861900 for all information.*

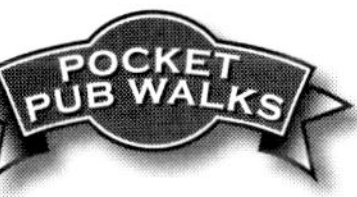

14 Sulgrave

The Star Inn

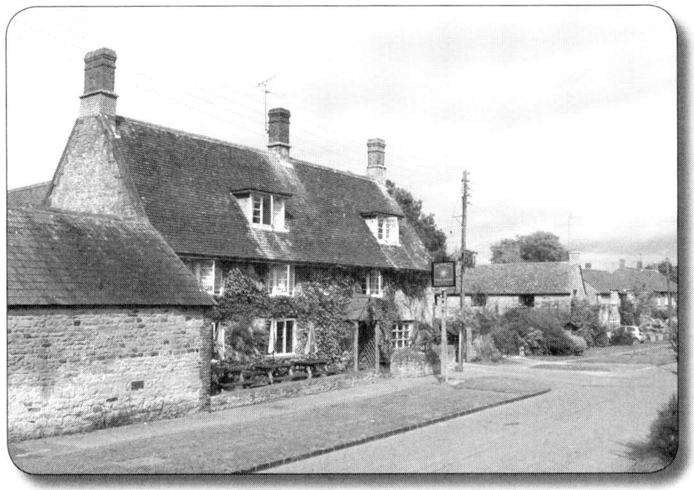

Sulgrave is an interesting village with some lovely old houses built of locally quarried stone. Its main claim to fame today is that Sulgrave Manor was the home of Lawrence Washington, a distant ancestor of the first President of the United States.

This lovely walk through undulating wooded countryside with beautiful views opening up takes you to the interesting village of Culworth before returning to Sulgrave across the fields and through a Site of Special Scientific Interest.

Distance – 4 miles.

OS Explorer 206 Edgehill & Fenny Compton. GR 557454.

Starting point The Star Inn in Manor Road. Customers may park here while they are walking – please ask first. There is also some roadside parking nearby.

How to get there *Sulgrave is west of the A43 near Towcester. Follow signs to Wappenham and Helmdon and thereafter to Sulgrave.*

THE PUB

What better way to enjoy a meal than sitting under a grapevine? That, among other things, is on offer at the 300-year-old **Star Inn**, which has a small bar area with an inglenook fireplace as well as a restaurant and, of course, the garden. Baguettes and sandwiches are on offer along with some very mouth-watering main courses, such as lemongrass and sundried tomato risotto or steak and sage sausages. There is also a 'Lite Bites' menu. The local Hooky Billet and Old Hooky ales are served alongside Carlsberg and Stella lagers and Guinness. Booking a table is advisable.

Food is available at lunchtime from 12 noon to 2 pm on Monday to Friday and 11.30 am to 2.30 pm at weekends; in the evening it is served from 6.30 pm to 9 pm on Monday to Friday, 6 pm to 10 pm on Saturday and 6.30 pm to 8.30 pm on Sunday.
☎ *01295 760389*

1 Turn right out of the pub along this pretty road of stone cottages and then go right down **Stockwell Lane** beside the little stone village shop and post office. Carry on along the lane until the

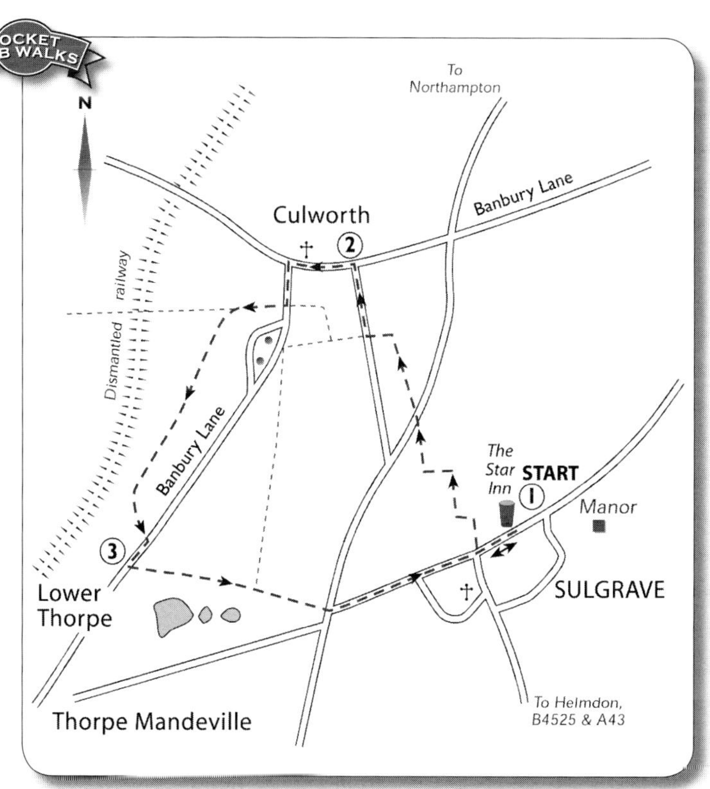

way is barred at the old watermill and turn left onto a track at the bottom of an amazing garden. The site has been landscaped and a mass of trees planted, some of them very rare, and ponds dug, spanned by exotic bridges. Continue up and round the garden, soon passing an organic orchard planted with apples, pears, plums, quinces and walnuts, which is owned by the Muslim mystic Sufi sect. Ahead lies the sight of a former windmill (now a private house) in front of which the road bends up to

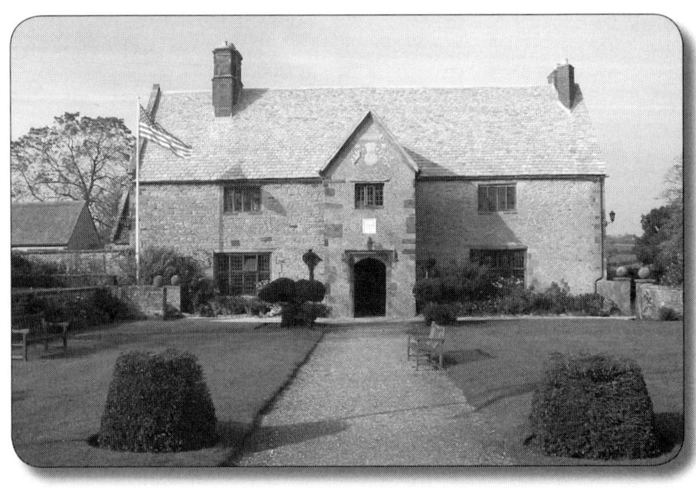

The 'Stars & Stripes' flies outside Sulgrave Manor.

the left. Just after a second safety mirror on the right there is gateway with a waymarker leading you across the field. Follow the markers over the road to a second road, at which point turn right into the village of **Culworth**. All is peace and quiet now but in the 18th century the notorious 'Culworth Gang' terrorised the area on the highways with cattle rustling and general thievery!

2 Walk along the village street, noticing a rather impressive stone arch over the entrance to **Culworth House** on the left. After passing the end of the churchyard, turn left down **Banbury Lane** and right opposite an oriental rug shop onto a concrete path. Just past the playing field, and at the end of a stone wall, turn left into a large field. Cross the field, going slightly right and down to a gap in the hedge over a little brook, then across the next field, aiming right of an oak tree to a small gap in the hedge. Continue across up to a farmyard and pick up a waymarker on a metal gate at the other end of the yard beside a small red brick

barn. At the bottom of the field go over a stile beside a wooden gate and follow the marker leading round the edge of the field to a metal gate with a stile beside it just short of the farm railings. Emerge onto **Banbury Lane**.

3 The next marker is well hidden behind the hedge opposite – so, turn right and then left up a drive and immediately left to a metal gate. Follow the path up the hill to the hedge to the right of a row of barns, carrying on until you arrive at a farm and go through the hedge onto the road. Here the route is well signed to **Sulgrave**. About 50 yards along this road on the left there is a wooden gate taking you onto the other side of the hedge for a pleasant walk back to the village (or if muddy carry on along the road into Sulgrave). An information board here makes interesting reading about the ecology of the area. Return to the road at the end of the hedge, continuing into the village and passing the stocks, which are quite unusual in that they also have two whipping posts. They have been heavily restored, hopefully not for present use. Return along the road to the **Star Inn**.

Place of interest nearby

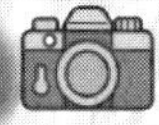

Sulgrave Manor in the village is certainly a 'must'. After the Dissolution of the Monasteries in 1539, Lawrence Washington bought the manor and his descendents lived there for 120 years. It was restored by the Anglo American Peace Committee and opened in 1921. It is a charming house to visit with Tudor to Georgian furniture as well as memorabilia. All manner of event days take place here, often with guides in clothes of the period. There is a shop and tearoom.

☎ *01295 760205 for details of opening times.*

POCKET PUB WALKS

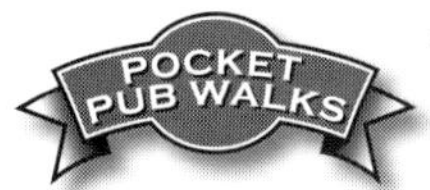

15 King's Sutton

The Butcher's Arms

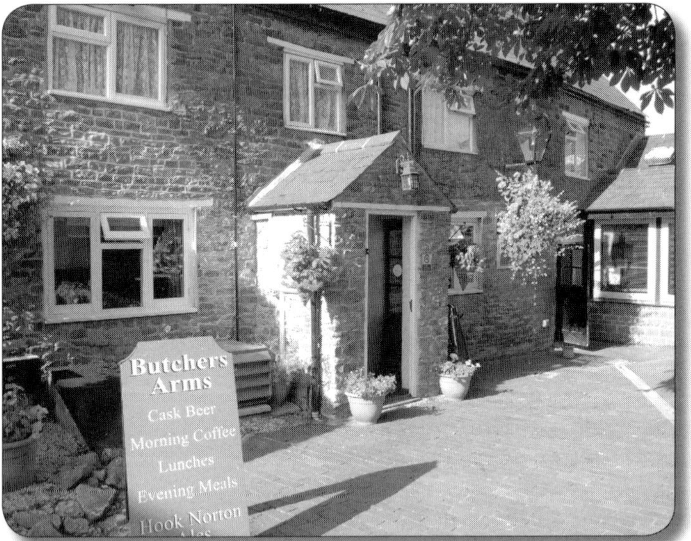

King's Sutton is one of those quintessential English villages; at its centre there is a large green with mature trees and stocks with the magnificent church of St Peter and St Paul at one end. The crocketed spire is so elegant and beautiful that it is reckoned to be one of the great spires of Northamptonshire. At one end of the village is an area known as Astrop Wells where people once came to take the waters for their medicinal properties. This was always done amid great merriment and feasting so one wonders how many went on their way actually the worse for wear!

The walk takes you across fields to the 'apricot' village of Aynho, with wonderful views of the Cherwell valley.

Distance – 3½ miles.

OS Explorer 191 Banbury, Bicester & Chipping Norton. GR 498362.

Starting point The Butcher's Arms is in Whittall Street, which runs north from the green at the opposite end from the church. The pub is about 30 yards down the hill on the right. There is a car park for patrons, otherwise one can park beside the road.

How to get there *Turn west off the A43 south of Brackley and follow signs to Charlton and King's Sutton.*

THE PUB The **Butcher's Arms** is a very nice pub which has a cosy oak-beamed bar area with an inglenook fireplace containing a wood-burning stove. There is a large dining room and, for good weather, picnic tables are set out in the garden at the back or under the magnificent chestnut tree in the front. The menu is small though varied because everything is home-cooked and is to be thoroughly recommended. The 'light bites' menu offers soup, filled baguettes, jacket potatoes and garlic mushrooms, amongst other things. The main menu offers chilli con carne, very succulent home-cooked ham as well as vegetarian dishes, and the excellent steak and ale pie will be enough to keep you walking for another three miles. There is also a grilled steak menu which is very comprehensive. This is a Hook Norton pub where there is a large selection of their beers along with John Smith's, Carling, Guinness, Stella and cider from the Stowford Press.

Food served Monday to Saturday from 12 noon to 2.30 pm and from 6.30 pm to 8.30 pm. A Sunday roast is served from 12 noon to 2.30 pm and 7 pm to 8.30 pm.
Tel. 01295 810898

1 On leaving the pub, turn left and left again onto **Astrop Road** and continue past a playing field. Just beyond where the road comes in from Middleton Cheney, turn right down a bridleway to **Walton Grounds** and at the end of the track bear right over a

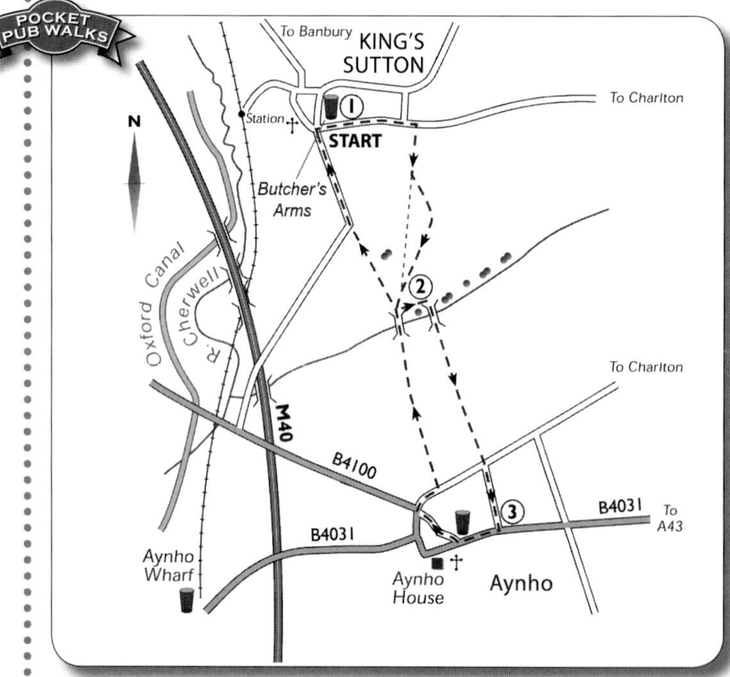

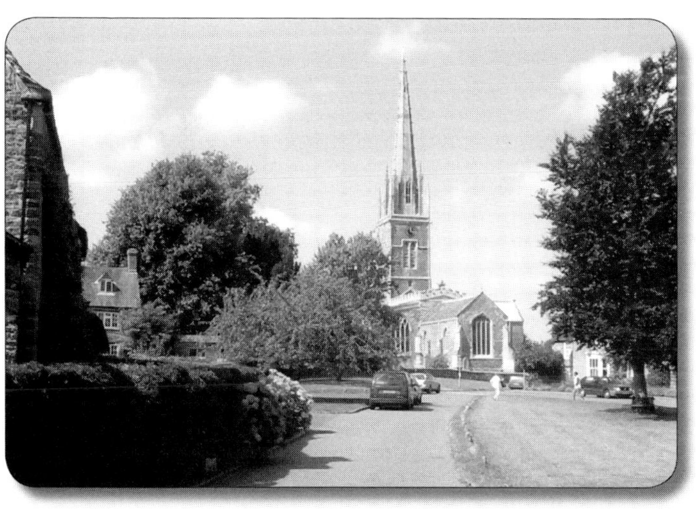

The church of St Peter and St Paul, with its crocketed spire.

metal gate and left along the path, keeping the hedge to the left. At a waymarker, carry on up the hill until you come to a footpath leading across the field to the right (there is no marker, but the farmer has left an obvious track) and cross diagonally to a row of trees. Go over the ditch and then diagonally left across the field, keeping left of a spinney in the centre.

2 Go through a gap in the hedge, following a sign diagonally right towards some houses. In the bottom right-hand corner, proceed down a narrow path with a private garden on the left and emerge onto a track. Turn left in front of two red brick houses, keeping a line of poplars on the right. After about 200 yards, veer right down to a gap in the hedge, cross the stream on a wooden bridge and continue up the hill, passing some farm sheds on the right. Halfway up the hill a thoughtful person has placed a bench so that you can sit and enjoy the lovely panorama. Carry on and

when reaching the road continue down **The Portway** (an old name for a road that linked villages together allowing people to go from market to market).

3 Just before the main road, turn right onto a paved footpath running between a stone wall and gardens. Then go left onto the pavement to follow the main road past the **Old Grammar School** and the **Cartwright Arms** in the middle of **Aynho**. This is known as the village of apricots and you will see them growing on the walls of many of the beautiful old stone cottages. Follow the main road round and downhill, passing **Aynho House**, once the seat of the Cartwright family but now separate dwellings. Halfway down the hill turn right into **Charlton Road** and in a short while turn left over a stone step stile into a field and then right to a gap in the hedge. Here a wonderful view opens up of the **Cherwell valley** through which run three examples of man's engineering ability: the Oxford Canal, the Great Western Railway and the M40 motorway (they ***are*** in the distance). Go on your way with the spire of **King's Sutton** before you, following through a gap in the hedge, taking the path right and then left. At the bottom of the path follow a sign leading right over the field to meet a track. Go straight ahead with **Twyford Farms** on the right. Continue along the road to a junction and a sign to **King's Sutton**. A sign with a charming raised stone flowerbed welcomes you back to the village.

Place of interest nearby

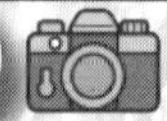

South-west of Banbury, the stunning moated **Broughton Castle**, completed in 1554, is owned by Lord and Lady Saye and Sele. Beautiful gardens surround the building, which was used for *Shakespeare in Love* among other films, and there is a lot to see and admire. The roses are a wonderful sight, especially in July. There is a shop, as well as a tearoom. ☎ *01295 276070.*